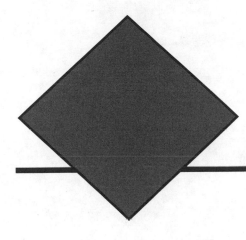

Examination Preparation

A Complete Guide for the
Physical Therapist Assistant

Scott M. Giles M.S., P.T.

Clinical Associate Professor
Department of Physical Therapy
University of New England
Biddeford, Maine

Ronda Sanders M.Ed., C.E.T.

Assistant Professor
Department of Learning Assistance and Individual Learning
University of New England
Biddeford, Maine

Mainely Physical Therapy
P.O. Box 7242
Scarborough, Maine 04070-7242

Toll Free: (866) PTEXAMS
Phone: (207) 885-0304
Fax: (207) 883-8377
Web site: www.ptexams.com

Acknowledgments

My sincere thanks to Therese Giles
and Gwenn Hoyt for their
valuable assistance with this project

Love to Traci, Meghan, Erin, Alexander, and Zachary

Special thanks to the many students who have
served as a constant source of inspiration

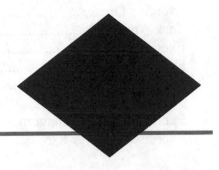

Table of Contents

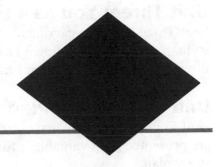

Introduction

The word examination can strike fear and anxiety into individuals like few other words in the English language. What is it about an examination that is so threatening to the majority of the population? The American Heritage Dictionary defines the word examination as "a set of questions designed to test knowledge." Although students are frequently exposed to examinations throughout their academic training, the thought of a comprehensive examination can make even the sturdiest student begin to perspire.

For physical therapist assistants, the ultimate comprehensive examination is the Physical Therapist Assistant Examination. The national examination serves to measure the knowledge and skills necessary for minimal competency as a physical therapist assistant and is often the final hurdle a physical therapist assistant must clear before obtaining licensure.

Perhaps a candidate's apprehension can be more clearly understood when viewing the significance of this examination. Candidates, in most cases, have recently completed their academic preparation and are eager to embark on their professional careers. They recognize that failure to meet or exceed the minimum scoring requirement on the examination can act as a barrier prohibiting them from practicing as a professional.

Our text is designed to maximize a candidate's performance on the Physical Therapist Assistant Examination. The text will accomplish this goal by taking candidates through eight distinct and separate units.

Unit One: Physical Therapist Assistant Examination
Unit One provides indepth information on the Physical Therapist Assistant Examination. It outlines the purpose, format, and design of the examination and addresses issues ranging from registration to scoring.

Unit Two: Time Management
Unit Two allows candidates to assess their time management skills. Candidates are presented with useful guidelines to consider when designing a study schedule.

Unit Three: You as a Learner

Unit Three provides candidates with the opportunity to assess their individual learning style. Candidates are shown how this information can be utilized as they prepare for the Physical Therapist Assistant Examination.

Unit Four: Study Plan

Unit Four explores the many different components of an effective study plan. Candidates are presented with valuable information to guide them as they develop an individualized study plan.

Unit Five: Multiple Choice Examinations

Unit Five analyzes the various components of a multiple choice examination. Suggested techniques to assist candidates when analyzing multiple choice questions are introduced. Candidates are given the opportunity to refine their test taking skills by answering selected examination questions.

Unit Six: Content Outline

Unit Six provides candidates with the opportunity to explore the content outline of the Physical Therapist Assistant Examination. A summary of each of the categories within the content outline is provided along with selected sample questions.

Unit Seven: Final Preparation

Unit Seven discusses issues for candidates to consider on the final days prior to the Physical Therapist Assistant Examination. Specific strategies to maximize performance and limit anxiety are discussed.

Unit Eight: Sample Examination

Unit Eight consists of a sample 150 question examination. Candidates are given the opportunity to refine their test taking skills and to assess their level of preparedness for the actual examination.

Physical Therapist Assistant Examination

The Physical Therapist Assistant Examination is a 175 question, multiple choice examination. The examination is designed to determine if candidates possess the minimal competency necessary to practice as physical therapist assistants.

The examination is created under the auspices of the Federation of State Boards of Physical Therapy. According to the National Physical Therapy Examination Candidate Handbook, the examination program serves two important purposes:

1. Provide examination services to authorities charged with the regulation of physical therapists and physical therapist assistants.

2. Provide a common element in evaluation of candidates so that standards will be comparable from jurisdiction to jurisdiction.

Registration

Registration occurs at the state level through the Physical Therapy State Licensing Agencies. The address of each agency, phone number, and web site are provided in the Appendix. Some state licensing agencies now permit online registration through the Federation of State Boards of Physical Therapy. Eligibility requirements vary considerably from jurisdiction to jurisdiction; therefore it is imperative that candidates carefully read all application information.

A variety of items may be required as part of the application process. These items may include a photograph; a notarized birth certificate; an official transcript from an accredited school; professional reference letters; and a check or money order for the required application, examination, and licensing fees.

It cannot be emphasized enough, however, that individual state licensing agencies' requirements vary. One small example is that many states will not accept any form of payment other than a money order or a certified bank check. If an applicant uses another form of payment, such as a personal check, the application could be considered incomplete. To avoid such difficulties, it is prudent to read the application carefully and to inquire as to the status of the application approximately two weeks after the completed application has been submitted.

Some states offer candidates with verifiable employment the opportunity to practice prior to being licensed by issuing a temporary license. Typically, candidates are required to have a completed application on file and have met all other qualifications for licensure before being considered for the temporary license. Temporary licenses are usually revoked if a candidate receives notification he/she was not successful on the Physical Therapist Assistant Examination.

Licensure

There are two primary ways in which to obtain a license to practice as a physical therapist assistant. They are termed examination and endorsement.

Examination
Licensure by examination is obtained after a candidate meets or exceeds the minimum scoring requirement on the Physical Therapist Assistant Examination and has satisfied all other state requirements. This form of obtaining licensure is the traditional method for candidates seeking initial licensure.

Endorsement
Licensure by endorsement using the Federation of State Boards of Physical Therapy Score Transfer Service makes it possible for candidates who have been licensed in a state by virtue of an examination to potentially gain licensure in another state without retaking the examination. Examination scores can be transferred to any physical therapy state licensing agency via the Federation of State Boards of Physical Therapy Score Transfer Service. The web site address for the Federation of State Boards of Physical Therapy is available in the Appendix.

Foreign Trained Therapists
Foreign trained therapists are subjected to a myriad of requirements before they are eligible to become licensed in the United States as a physical therapist or physical therapist assistant. Since the requirements vary significantly by state, it is recommended that candidates contact the physical therapy state licensing agency within the state they intend to practice. The state licensing agency can provide detailed information on their individual requirements.

There are two general requirements that seem to be consistent in all states for foreign trained therapists:

1. Applicants are required to submit their educational credentials for evaluation of their equivalence to the United States trained applicant.

2. Applicants must meet or exceed the minimum scoring requirements on the Physical Therapist Examination or the Physical Therapist Assistant Examination.

Other state requirements can include, but are not limited to, the following:

- Demonstrate proficiency in written and spoken English
- Submit letters of reference
- Obtain a valid visa and resident alien card
- Complete an internship or period of supervised practice
- Appear for an interview
- Attain the equivalent of a United States grade of "C" or higher in all professional coursework

Examination Development

According to the Federation of State Boards of Physical Therapy, the Physical Therapist Assistant Examination is developed by three committees. These committees are the Examination Construction and Review Committee; the Item Bank Review Committee; and the Item Writer Regional Coordinators.

The Examination Construction and Review Committee is responsible for determining the content categories and subcategories of the examination and the percentage of items in each area. The categories are based on the tasks and roles performed by physical therapist assistants. The information necessary to create each category and subcategory is obtained after analyzing the responses of hundreds of physical therapist assistants to a job analysis survey. The most recent job analysis survey occurred in 2001 and was introduced in the new content outline in November of 2002. The content outline is typically revised on a five year cycle.

Individual physical therapists and physical therapist assistants have direct involvement in writing examination questions. The therapists involved are required to attend item-writing workshops that are taught by experienced testing professionals. Questions, once completed, are analyzed independently to make sure they are reflective of the current examination content outline. The focus of the examination questions is on problem solving and away from rote memorization of fact. Candidates are required to demonstrate their ability to apply knowledge in a safe and effective manner.

Examination Administration

Candidates begin the application process by obtaining a general application form and a computerized scannable information form from a physical therapy state licensing agency. Once completed, the forms are returned along with any necessary fees to the state licensing agency. After a candidate's application is approved, the state licensing agency forwards the computerized form to the Federation of State Boards of Physical Therapy. A limited number of states are now permitting candidates to apply online through the Federation of State Boards of Physical Therapy.

The Federation of State Boards of Physical Therapy issues candidates an "approval to test" letter that includes instructions on how to schedule an appointment to take the examination. Candidates must sit for the examination within 60 days of the date on their letter. The examination is offered on computer at over 300 Prometric Testing Centers within the United States or at selected testing facilities in Canada. Testing is offered Monday through Saturday from 9:00 AM - 6:00 PM. Within each Prometric Testing Center candidates can concentrate on the examination without environmental distracters. Private, modular booths provide adequate work space with proper lighting and ventilation. All Prometric Testing Centers are fully accessible.

Candidates are not limited to the testing centers within the state they are applying for licensure. For example, a student that has recently graduated from a physical therapy program in Maine could apply for licensure in California and take the required examination while still in Maine.

It is important to note that basic computer skills are not necessary with computer based testing. Prior to beginning the examination, candidates utilize a tutorial which explains topics such as selecting answers and navigating within the examination. Time spent on the computer tutorial does not count towards the allotted time for the actual examination.

Candidates have the option of entering their answers using a computer keyboard or mouse. Once within the actual examination candidates can move freely between examination questions. Candidates can go back to previously answered or unanswered questions and make any desired changes. Candidates are allowed to use scratch paper supplied by the testing center during the examination.

Content Outline

The content outline provides candidates with a detailed description of the information contained on the Physical Therapist Assistant Examination. Although listed here, the content outline will be discussed in detail in Unit Six.

Federation of State Boards of Physical Therapy

Physical Therapist Assistant Examination

I. **Tests and Measures (Data Collection)**
   Tests and Measures Group I
   1. Strength, ROM, Posture, Body Structures
   2. Cognition, Reflex and Sensory Integrity

   Tests and Measures Group II
   1. Cardiovascular/pulmonary System – endurance, circulation, physiological status, ventilation, respiration tests
   2. Integumentary System – observe patient skin status; observe and measure patient wounds (e.g. size, depth)
   3. Functional Status – assistive and adaptive devices, gait, balance, pain, body mechanics

II. **Intervention**
   Non-procedural Interventions
   1. Coordination of care
   2. Interpersonal communication
   3. Documentation
   4. Patient/family/client-related instructions

   Procedural Interventions
   Group I: Exercise and manual therapy

   Group II: Transfer and functional activities, gait training, assistive and adaptive devices, and modification of the environment

   Group III: Physical agents and modalities

   Group IV: Airway clearance techniques, wound care, promoting health and wellness, and intervention effectiveness

III. **Standards of Care**
   A. Patient confidentiality, autonomy, and consent
   B. Work Parameters
   1. Work under the direction and supervision of a PT in an ethical, legal, safe, and effective manner
   2. Knowing and working within state law and rules governing physical therapy

3. Performing only those tasks that are within the PTAs knowledge and skill level
4. Utilizing clinical decision making in data collection and interventions
C. Body mechanics/positioning/draping
D. Safety, CPR, emergency care, first aid
E. Standard precautions

Scoring

The actual Physical Therapist Assistant Examination is 175 questions, however 25 of the questions serve as pretest items and are not officially scored. The pretest items allow new examination questions to be evaluated throughout the year and eliminate lengthy delays in score reporting. Candidates are unable to differentiate between pretest and scored items on the 175 question examination. To accommodate for the increased number of questions, candidates receive an additional 30 minutes to complete the examination. Candidates have a total of 3.5 hours to complete the 175 question examination. Since candidate performance is based solely on the number of scored items answered correctly, the sample examination in Unit Eight consists of only 150 questions.

The Federation of State Boards of Physical Therapy is responsible for scoring the examination and reporting results to the individual state licensing agencies. The state licensing agencies then notify candidates as to their performance on the examination. Formal notification typically occurs through the mail, however many state licensing agencies have web sites that allow candidates to determine their licensing status online. In most instances, candidates' scores are available within 3-10 days.

The questions are multiple choice with four possible answers to each question. Candidates are asked to identify the best answer to each of the questions. Each question has only one correct answer. A candidate's score is determined based on the number of questions answered correctly. Candidates accumulate one point for each correctly answered question. There is no penalty for questions answered incorrectly. The total cumulative score is termed the total raw score. The maximum total raw score for the Physical Therapist Assistant Examination is 150.

Criterion-referenced scoring is used to determine passing scores on the Physical Therapist Assistant Examination. Passing scores are determined based on the judgment of selected experts on the minimum number of questions that should be answered correctly by a minimally qualified candidate. Criterion-referenced passing scores are determined independently of candidate performance and are designed to reflect the difficulty of each examination. For example, if a given examination was judged to be particularly difficult, the minimum passing score would be lower than another examination that was judged to be less difficult.

Since the minimum passing score is based on the difficulty of the examination, it becomes impossible to determine an automatic passing score. Historically, criterion-referenced passing scores have ranged from 102 - 114. If the criterion-referenced passing score was established as 110 for a given examination, a total raw score of greater than or equal to 110 would be considered a passing score, while a total raw score of less than 110 would be considered a failing score. Within a given examination cycle, criterion-referenced passing scores usually fluctuate in a much smaller range, perhaps by as few as five questions.

An individual examination score is often reported to candidates in the form of a scaled score. Scaled scores range from 200 - 800 with the minimum passing score always being equal to a scaled score of 600. Scaled scores are necessary as a method of equating examinations with different criterion-referenced passing scores.

If a candidate is successful on the examination, in most cases they have fulfilled the final requirement for licensure. Conversely, if a candidate is unsuccessful on the examination, they are required to reapply to the state licensing agency. With computer based testing there is no mandatory waiting period before retaking the examination, however some states limit the number of times a candidate can take the examination or mandate remedial coursework.

Candidates that were unsuccessful on the Physical Therapist Assistant Examination can elect to receive role feedback. The role feedback report compares individual examination performance with that of other candidates taking the same examination. Additional information on role feedback is available through the Federation of State Boards of Physical Therapy.

In addition to the Physical Therapist Assistant Examination, a number of states also require candidates to successfully complete a jurisprudence examination. This type of examination is based on the state rules and regulations governing physical therapy practice. The examination can include multiple choice items, short answer questions, or fill in the blanks. States can administer the examination using computer based testing or even as a take home examination.

Coming Attractions

As you have progressed through this unit, you most likely have gained an appreciation for the complexity of preparing for the Physical Therapist Assistant Examination. Although this task can, at times, seem overwhelming there are a number of strategies that can significantly enhance a candidate's preparation efficiency and organization. These areas are:

- Time management skills
- A viable study plan

- Knowledge of how you learn
- Test taking skills

Each of these four areas will be discussed in detail in upcoming units. Candidates should attempt to apply the information obtained in these units as they prepare for the Physical Therapist Assistant Examination.

Time Management

Time management is, perhaps, the most overlooked component of a comprehensive study plan. Most candidates take the Physical Therapist Assistant Examination shortly after graduation. This can be a very anxious and unsettled time. Candidates often are actively seeking employment or are attempting to adjust to a new job. They may have relocated to a different residence or perhaps moved to another part of the country. To further complicate matters, they are starting to focus on the impending Physical Therapist Assistant Examination.

Time Management Assessment

Time management is not about meeting deadlines and getting things done. Time management is about keeping our lives in balance. We will classify the major areas of our lives into four distinct and separate categories. These areas are listed and defined below:

The emotional you: your inner self - your ongoing and ever-changing perceptions and reflections on life, self, values, etc.

The intellectual you: your intellectually curious self - student, reader, researcher, etc.

The physical you: your physical self - walking, running, swimming, grooming, etc.

The social you: your outer self - social interactions with family, friends, church activities, etc.

When the balance among these four areas is disturbed, stress inevitably results. One of the major by-products of stress is the inability to concentrate and retain information. Failure to concentrate while preparing for a comprehensive examination such as the Physical Therapist Assistant Examination can have devastating results.

How balanced are your days? Find out by keeping an Activity Log for a three day period. A sample Activity Log is located in the Appendix. Attempt to follow your normal daily routine during these three days. At the end of each day, summarize your activity using the Time Management Diagnostic Sheet.

Time Management Diagnostic Sheet

	Day One	Day Two	Day Three	Total
CLASS				
STUDY				
INDIVIDUAL TIME				
SOCIAL TIME				
EXERCISE				
WORK				
SLEEP				
NAP				
NIGHT				
SPECIAL APPOINTMENT				

After completing the diagnostic activity sheet, attempt to determine how balanced your days are. Ask yourself if there are any of the four areas of your life that are not represented in your daily activities. If deficient areas are identified, attempt to select activities to augment these areas.

Are you getting some physical activity? A twenty minute walk may be sufficient. Did you find time, or did you simply not get around to it? Was it too cold out, or did you simply not feel like exercising?

How about your social self? These times include social functions, conversations with friends and family, or non-working lunches. Did you avoid others because you were not feeling very sociable, or did you feel you had too much to do without wasting time playing?

Did you nurture your emotional self? This reflective area of life is the most diverse among people, and often the most neglected. Some people serve their emotional needs in church, some like to meditate or listen to music. Did you avoid such activities because you felt you simply did not have the time to spare or did you feel it was relatively unimportant with all of your other pressing needs?

How about intellectual stimulation? Probably at this point your intellectual self is being pandered to for many hours each day preparing for the examination. However, it is healthy to have a few other intellectual pursuits not related to the examination. Have you placed other intellectual pursuits like reading the newspaper or watching the news on hold because you are immersed in preparing for the examination with every waking moment?

Candidates also need to assess their ability to concentrate. Do you find yourself drifting off and glancing at the clock to discover that twenty minutes has elapsed and you have no idea where the time went? Do you feel that your study breaks seem to get longer as your study session progresses? Do you elect not to take study breaks and find yourself waking up in the cold, early hours of the morning, slumped over your books with a sore neck? Can you find a million "necessary" chores to do in order to avoid settling down to study?

If you answered yes to any of the preceding questions, you may benefit from improved time management. Remember, stress is progressive, so the ability to concentrate and retain information will decrease as time goes on. We suggest that you try the following two-part program.

Time Management Program

Part One: Long-Range Planning

Step 1: Find a calendar and identify the months between now and when you plan to take the examination.

Step 2: Use the content outline and begin to assign time to each of the three content areas so that they can be reviewed adequately prior to the examination.

Since the three content areas vary significantly in their weighting, it is imperative that candidates also weight the study time dedicated to each area. The specific weighting of each of the content areas is discussed in detail in Unit Six.

A sample two-month, long-range schedule is illustrated below:

Sample Two Month Long-Range Schedule

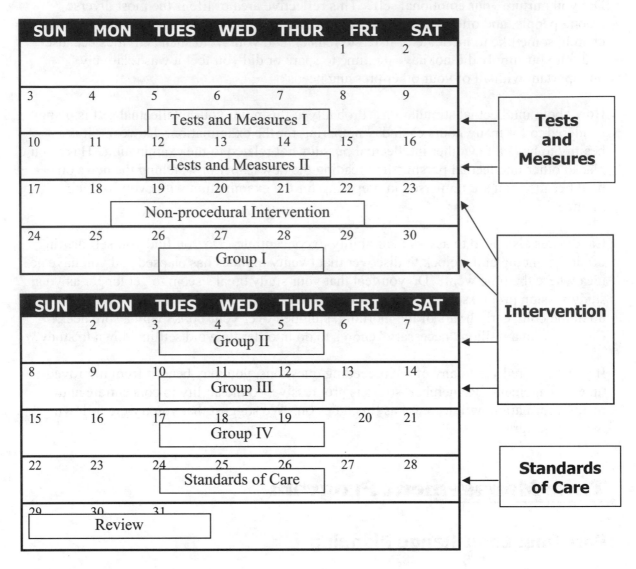

Part Two: Weekly Planning

Step 1: Assign a color to each of the four areas of your life: emotional, intellectual, physical, and social.

Step 2: Develop a master weekly schedule that includes all of your scheduled activities. These activities can include items such as: study sessions, work, church, social engagements, and exercise sessions. Mark each of the activities that appear on the master schedule with the appropriate color.

Step 3:   Determine which, if any, of the four areas is being neglected in your present schedule. Select activities that can augment the deficient areas and assign them times, keeping in mind the following:

Emotional: Individual reflection time allocated for thinking about issues important to you; done independently, goal-directed, resolution-oriented, time-limited; most people plan for one half-hour, or two fifteen minute periods daily, neither just before bed.

Intellectual: Involves study time or clinical practice; follow the study plan suggested for your learning style, taking into consideration your learning environment preferences (Unit Three).

Physical: Works best if not done immediately after a meal or just before bedtime; combines well with emotional or social time immediately afterwards.

Social: Includes meal time, movies, theater, etc; works best when scheduled before a firm commitment, since individuals are most likely to lose track of time in this area.

Step 4:   Complete the schedule, being sure to leave at least one hour each day unfilled. When a scheduled activity is missed, it can be rescheduled easily within the available time.

Step 5:   Follow the schedule for at least one week and then do a self-assessment of your satisfaction with your productivity and concentration during study times. You may find it necessary to make adjustments to your future schedule based on your progress.

The following table illustrates a sample weekly schedule, which has been coded to correspond to each of the four areas of your life. By quickly examining the schedule, it becomes fairly easy to determine the relative weighting of each area. Candidates should attempt to design an individual schedule that is consistent with their present life status.

Sample Weekly Time Management Schedule

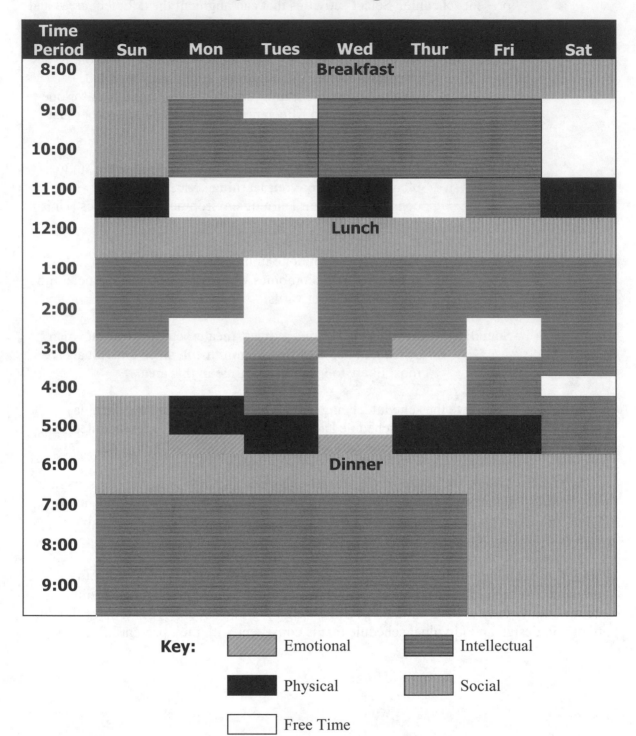

Time Period	Sun	Mon	Tues	Wed	Thur	Fri	Sat
8:00				Breakfast			
9:00							
10:00							
11:00							
12:00				Lunch			
1:00							
2:00							
3:00							
4:00							
5:00							
6:00				Dinner			
7:00							
8:00							
9:00							

Key:

Emotional   Intellectual

Physical   Social

Free Time

You as a Learner

We imagine that at some time during your college years, you have observed the most obnoxious learner of all, the one who never seems to study and then consistently receives an "A" on every examination. This person does not necessarily have any more intelligence than other students, but simply may have developed a sense of how he/she learns most efficiently and is therefore able to develop a study plan based on his/her individual learning needs. It is our hope that the time management strategies presented earlier, in combination with the material that will be conveyed in this unit, will enable you to develop an efficient and effective individualized study plan.

To discover how you function as a learner, you need to answer three specific questions:

1. What combination of the three learning channels do you prefer for input and processing?
2. What is your dominant thinking mode?
3. What is your optimum learning environment?

The Three Learning Channels

There are three basic ways of perceiving information: see it (visual), hear it (auditory), or be physically involved in doing it (tactile/kinesthetic). The combination of these channels that an individual uses, both the first time he/she is exposed to new material (input) and during subsequent exposure (processing), determines one of the facets of learning style. Each individual's preference of channels for input and processing determines Active/Passive learning patterns.

Attempt to classify your preferred learning style for input and processing into one of the following four categories:

Active/Active

If you are an individual who, the first time you are exposed to new material likes to hear it, see it, say it, question it, interact with it, and then keep right on doing this, you would be categorized as a multisensoral (visual, auditory, and tactile/kinesthetic) active learner for both input and processing. These individuals immediately attempt to determine the relevance and utility of material and must, at input, be able to relate it to previous knowledge or experience. They typically find it difficult, and sometimes impossible, to go into a room alone, open up a book, and read.

Strengths:

- focus on application and utility of ideas
- 100% concentration on activities for short periods of time
- flexibility and adaptability

Weaknesses:

- may consider details boring
- short attention span may lead to incomplete preparation
- high distractibility may disrupt concentration

Active/Passive

If you are an individual who, the first time you are exposed to new material, likes to hear it, see it, say it, question it, interact with it, and then take a visual reference home to study by yourself, you would be classified as a multisensoral learner for input and a visual processor. These individuals need to relate new material, at input, to previous knowledge or experience.

Strengths:

- focus on gathering extensive data
- long-term memory
- strong visual channel often allows them to visualize notes, text, charts in their mind's eye

Weaknesses:

- may not focus on utility or use of information
- may require more time to learn new material
- may have a tendency to gather excessive information in an area of special interest and neglect other important areas

Passive/Active

If you are an individual who, the first time you are exposed to new material, likes either to hear it in lecture form or to read it in a book, and then utilize the material in an interactive way (visual, auditory, tactile/kinesthetic), you would be categorized as a passive learner for input and an active processor. These individuals relate new material to previous knowledge or experience and determine the relevance and utility of the material after input and before processing.

Strengths:

- focus on both facts/concepts and clinical application
- synthesis of known information into a plan of action
- sequential and relational thought

Weaknesses:

- may have difficulty determining proportional importance of information
- may begin applying information before sufficient details have been gathered
- may fail to identify the relationship to previous knowledge or experience

Passive/Passive

If you are an individual who, the first time you are exposed to new material, likes either to hear it or to read it and prefers to keep right on doing that, you would be categorized as a passive learner for both input and processing. These individuals determine the relationship to known material after input and before processing.

Strengths:

- sequential thinking
- focus on details
- strong visual channel that allows one to visualize notes, text, charts in their mind's eye

Weaknesses:

- may miss the "big picture"
- may have difficulty answering application questions requiring relational thinking
- tendency to study alone often inhibits opportunities to examine information from different perspectives

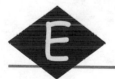

Exercise One

Once you have identified your preferred learning style for input and processing, attempt to classify the strength of your preference. We have divided this category into slight, decided and strong.

If all of the descriptors in one of the categories describe your learning style, place a check under strong preference. If the majority, but not all of the descriptors were accurate, place a check next to decided. If a few more of the descriptors in one category, when compared to the others, describe your learning style, place a check next to slight.

The stronger one's preference for a specific category, the less flexible a candidate will be in his/her input and processing channel needs. Candidates with a strong preference will need to pay particular attention to the recommendations for their learning style in Unit Four.

Input/Processing Preferences

	Slight	Decided	Strong
Active/Active	☐	☐	☐
Active/Passive	☐	☐	☐
Passive/Active	☐	☐	☐
Passive/Passive	☐	☐	☐

◆   ◆   ◆

Thinking Modes

You probably have heard the terms "left-brained" and "right-brained." In this book, these are not physiological or psychological terms, but instead educational terms which describe a set of learning characteristics. The following table depicts "left-brain" and "right-brain" learners' characteristics:

"Left" Thinking	"Right" Thinking
Facts	"What if.....?"
Words	Pictures
Sequences	Relationships
Details	Global concepts
Analytical	Synthetic

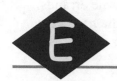

Exercise Two

Complete the following informal exercise to evaluate your thinking mode.

1. Look over the text and the chart. Both contain the same information. Assume you are attempting to learn the information for the first time and that you have no previous knowledge of fruits' shapes or colors.

Fruits come in many shapes and colors. Oranges, kiwi, and tangerines are round; bananas are oblong; and pears are "pear shaped."

Oranges and tangerines are orange; bananas and pears are yellow; a kiwi is green.

	Shape			Color		
	Round	Pear	Oblong	Orange	Yellow	Green
Oranges	•			•		
Tangerines	•			•		
Bananas			•		•	
Pears		•			•	
Kiwi	•					•

If you were more comfortable learning the information about fruit from the two paragraphs of text, place an **X** next to the "L" below. If the table appealed to you more, place an **X** next to the "R". If you are equally comfortable with both, place an **X** next to the "I" (integrated).

_____ "L"   _____ "I"   _____ "R"

2. Picture the following scenario: You are going downtown to do some errands. Your errands will require you to go to the bank, the post office, the hardware store, the gas station, and the grocery store. The location of each facility is as follows:

❖ **Bank**

❖ **Gas Station**

❖ **Grocery Store**

❖ **Hardware Store**

❖ **Post Office**

❖ **Your Home**

If, either before leaving the house or while you were driving, you would think about the sequence in which you plan to do the errands in the most efficient way, place an **X** next to the "L". If you would complete the errands in a random order, place an **X** next to the "R". If sometimes you would plan and sometimes you would not, place an **X** next to the "I".

_____ "L"   _____ "I"   _____ "R"

◆   ◆   ◆

Learning Environment

The following checklist, although by no means complete, can help you identify the learning environment best suited for your concentration and learning needs. Place a check mark in the boxes next to the items that you prefer.

Individual Preferences		
☐ Morning	☐ Afternoon	☐ Evening
☐ Quiet	☐ Soft Music	☐ Noisy
☐ Sitting	☐ Standing	☐ Moving
☐ Snacking	☐ Talking	☐ Writing
☐ Typing	☐ Colorful Room	☐ Muted Tones
☐ Alone	☐ Partner	☐ Group

Input/Processing Preferences			
Frequency of Meetings	☐ Regularly	☐ Often	☐ As Needed
Duration of Sessions	☐ One Hour	☐ Two Hours	☐ Flexible
Structure	☐ Hierarchical	☐ Participative	☐ Debate

Learning Profile Application

After progressing through the three learning style exercises, you may be wondering how this information can be utilized to assist you with your preparation for the Physical Therapist Assistant Examination. Each of the learning style activities provides unique insight into your individual learning style.

The knowledge acquired about your input and processing needs can be utilized as a guide to design your study schedule to suit your Active/Passive preferences. For example, if you have identified that you prefer to be active at input, you intentionally can incorporate visual, auditory, and/or tactile-kinesthetic stimulation into your study sessions. Let's assume that you are reviewing orthopedic special tests. The visual channel can be activated by reading orthopedic textbooks, examining pictures, or watching videotapes of selected special tests. The auditory channel can be activated by listening to yourself or others talk about selected special tests, and the tactile/kinesthetic channel can be utilized by performing selected special tests on another individual.

This same approach can be utilized regardless of the material being reviewed or relearned. It is probably not realistic for individuals to always plan learning experiences based solely on their learning style preferences; however, consistent use of a preferred learning style will tend to maximize a candidate's efficiency during his/her preparation for the Physical Therapist Assistant Examination.

The knowledge acquired about your learning environment preferences can assist you in creating a productive study atmosphere when working alone or with others. It also can assist you in selecting an appropriate study partner and/or indicate whether you are a good candidate for group learning.

The knowledge acquired about thinking mode preferences will apply directly to the questions on the Physical Therapist Assistant Examination. Since the examination emphasizes clinically oriented material, it requires integrated thinking. Candidates must not only know cognitive information, but they must also demonstrate performance proficiency. Suggestions for an effective information gathering system to achieve integration will be presented in Unit Five.

If you determined you were left-brain dominant on the thinking mode exercise, you probably will be more comfortable answering questions that demonstrate more of a left-brain bias. Conversely, if you are right-brain dominant, you probably will be more comfortable answering questions that demonstrate more of a right-brain bias. Examination questions, although usually requiring integrated thinking, still may have a left or right-brain bias. By being familiar with the characteristics of both left and right-brain questions, candidates can develop an increased awareness of their own learning style and develop particular learning activities directed toward their non-dominant thinking mode.

Sample Questions

The following section provides three sample questions. As you read each of the questions, take note of those which are easy for you and those which are more of a challenge, and see if you can determine why. A brief analysis of each question is presented, along with an answer key at the conclusion of the exercise.

Each of the answer keys throughout the text lists the best answer to each question and identifies a resource which supports the stated answer. In the vast majority of cases a page number is also provided to direct candidates to the appropriate subject matter. The complete reference for each of the resources is located in the bibliography.

Sample Question One:

A physical therapist assistant examines a patient that has burns over her anterior right arm, the anterior portion of the thorax, and the genital region. Based on the "rule of nines", what percentage of the patient's body is affected?

1. 19.0%
2. 22.5%
3. 23.5%
4. 28.0%

Analysis: This question will tend to favor left-brain dominant candidates. The question requires candidates to recall detailed information, specifically the percentage of the total body surface allocated to the nine various anatomical segments.

Sample Question Two:

A physical therapist assistant observes a patient ambulating in the physical therapy gym. The therapist notes that the patient's pelvis drops on the right during left stance phase. In an attempt to compensate, the patient laterally bends his trunk over the stance leg. This type of gait deviation can be caused by weakness of the:

1. gluteus maximus
2. gluteus medius
3. iliopsoas
4. tensor fasciae latae

Analysis: This question will tend to favor right-brain dominant candidates. The question requires candidates to identify the relationship between a specific muscle function and a resultant gait deviation.

Sample Question Three:

A physical therapist assistant is treating a six-month-old infant with spina bifida. The infant suddenly begins to act strangely during the treatment session. A primary survey reveals the infant is not breathing, but does have a pulse. The most immediate response would be to:

1. begin chest compressions
2. begin mouth to mouth breathing
3. begin mouth to nose breathing
4. begin mouth to mouth and nose breathing

Analysis: This question is more representative of the integrated type that will make up the majority of the Physical Therapist Assistant Examination. This specific question requires candidates not only to be familiar with the sequential steps of cardiopulmonary resuscitation, but also to recognize the relationship among a number of other factors including when a patient has a pulse and is not breathing. The candidate is further required to identify the most immediate response.

Answer Key

1. Answer: 3   Resource: O'Sullivan (p. 852)
   The percentage of the total body surface burned in an adult can be calculated using the rule of nines: anterior right arm 4.5%, anterior portion of the thorax 18%, genital region 1%. Total = 23.5%

2. Answer: 2   Resource: Magee (p. 866)
   The gluteus medius muscle is a hip abductor. Weakness of the abductor can result in a Trendelenburg gait.

3. Answer: 4   Resource: American Heart Association
                                                (p. 148)
   Mouth to mouth and nose breathing is utilized on an infant (less than one year).

As you progress through the sample questions in this text, it should become apparent that to be successful on the examination, a candidate will have to demonstrate both left and right-brain proficiency. It is therefore advisable for a candidate's study plan to incorporate activities which utilize both left-brain and right-brain thinking modes.

We will continue to expand on many of the topics we have introduced throughout the text. Included in the following unit will be general and specific study guidelines and specific learning style recommendations.

Study Plan

The simple thought of preparing for a comprehensive examination such as the Physical Therapist Assistant Examination can be overwhelming. Many candidates ask themselves how it is possible to prepare adequately for an examination that encompasses more than two years of professional coursework.

One of the largest advantages of taking an examination such as the Physical Therapist Assistant Examination is that it does not require candidates to demonstrate mastery of new material. On the surface this may not seem like a significant advantage, but since candidates are, in effect, only reviewing or relearning previously presented information, their level of attainment should be significantly greater.

Many candidates fail to utilize this advantage. Candidates who attempt to learn large quantities of new information, instead of focusing on understanding and applying basic concepts, often do themselves a tremendous disservice. It is true that there undoubtedly will be questions that contain information that was not part of a selected curriculum, but to attempt to study this new information in any significant detail would be a large mistake for most candidates. Instead, candidates should focus on reviewing or relearning basic concepts that are an integral component of all accredited physical therapist assistant programs. It is this type of information that will make up the vast majority of the examination. Individuals who take this common sense approach optimize their chances of success on this important examination.

Developing a Plan

Developing a study plan allows candidates to take control of their preparation. Candidates should begin by compiling a list of all the necessary topics that must be reviewed prior to the examination. The topics should be assembled in a sequence that will allow for a smooth transition between topics. Candidates should make an estimate of the time needed to review each topic and compile a list of available resources.

The Reporter's Formula

Throughout history, individuals have been sent out to gather information about ideas, events, processes, and people. To assist these individuals, a specific formula was developed. This formula was termed "the reporter's formula."

The reporter's formula contains the following seven question words: Who, What, Which, When, Where, How, and Why. This time tested technique of information gathering can be utilized by candidates preparing for the Physical Therapist Assistant Examination in a number of different ways:

1. Incorporate the formula into a study plan for each content category
2. Utilize the formula as an outline for study sessions
3. Generate potential examination questions using the formula

The formula also can be used to categorize actual examination questions. This specific technique will be explored in detail in Unit Five.

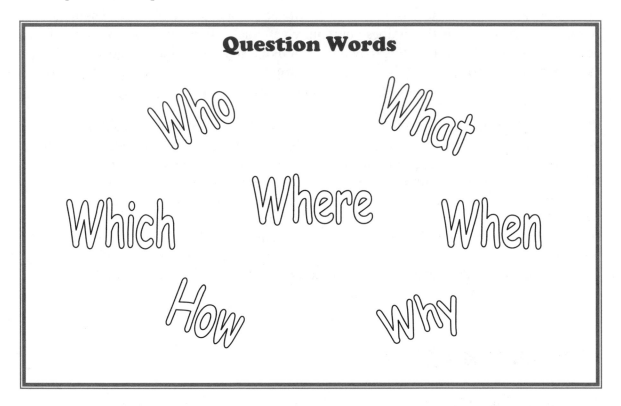

Goals

Before beginning to study, develop specific goals for each study session. Ideally, these goals should be established on a weekly basis. Establishing goals will ensure that candidates cover the desired material and will serve as a mechanism to keep them on schedule with their study plan. Candidates should be realistic with the goals they establish and should not attempt to cover more material than is possible in a particular study session.

Reviewing

Reviewing is defined operationally as looking over or studying previously learned information. Reviewing can play an important role in a candidate's preparation for the Physical Therapist Assistant Examination. It is recommended that students review classnotes for their practice oriented professional coursework. Practice oriented professional coursework typically includes, but is not limited to, study of the musculoskeletal, neuromuscular, cardiopulmonary, and integumentary systems. In addition, candidates usually have coursework in patient care skills, physical agents, administration, ethics, and education. Each of these topics are important components of the content outline for the Physical Therapist Assistant Examination.

Classnotes may seem voluminous to candidates, but they can be reviewed fairly quickly. Special attention must be taken not to become bogged down in one specific area for any significant amount of time. General concepts that are understood should be scanned quickly, while other concepts that are more difficult for a candidate should be read carefully. Concepts that remain unclear after being reviewed should be written down for future study sessions.

Other foundational coursework encountered earlier in the professional curriculum can be consulted as needed during various study sessions. This type of coursework often includes, but is not limited to Anatomy and Physiology, Neuroanatomy, Exercise Physiology, and Kinesiology. It is important to limit the amount of time spent reviewing this type of foundational coursework. Candidates often can make better use of their allotted time by reviewing coursework encountered later in the curriculum that may be more practice oriented. By reviewing practice oriented information, candidates not only keep their studying consistent with the format of the examination, but at the same time indirectly review much of the information presented in the foundational coursework.

Relearning

Relearning is defined operationally as reacquiring knowledge or comprehension which was known previously. Relearning is often a necessary component of a comprehensive study plan. In physical therapy academic programs, candidates constantly are learning new information on a variety of topics. Although students typically exhibit mastery of selected material during a scheduled examination, they do not always retain the information for later use. Failure to retain information that was learned previously is the primary rationale for relearning.

Relearning can take place in a variety of ways. Often times, simply reviewing information is enough for candidates to relearn the material; however, in some cases, a more indepth approach is necessary. This approach may include using textbooks, class handouts, and interacting with classmates or professors. It is imperative that candidates relearn material which may be an integral component of the examination. It must be stressed, however, that to focus on memorizing minuscule facts or inordinate details would be, at best, poor utilization of available study time.

Journal

It is recommended that candidates keep a daily journal of their studying. This journal should include a variety of information:

1. Topics/concepts that were reviewed successfully
2. Topics/concepts requiring additional review or relearning
3. List of goals for each study session
4. Progress towards meeting established goals
5. Resources utilized during the study session
6. Plan for the subsequent study session

As candidates begin to complete sample examinations, the journal will allow them to document specific information on their performance. This should include the percentage of questions answered correctly and the amount of time necessary to complete a selected examination. Candidates should survey questions that were answered incorrectly and attempt to determine if there are any general patterns. For example, if a candidate consistently has difficulty answering questions related to a specific topic area or questions that were constructed in a similar manner, these deficits should be recorded. Once identified, appropriate remedial strategies can be developed.

General Recommendations

To this point, candidates have learned a variety of strategies to utilize when developing a study plan for the Physical Therapist Assistant Examination. There are, however, a variety of other variables that can influence the quality of a study session. This text will describe many of these variables.

Environment

To construct an optimal learning environment, candidates should attempt to incorporate their individual learning preferences into each study session. Return to Unit Three to reexamine the preferences best suited for your specific concentration and learning needs.

Supplies

Gather the necessary supplies to assist you in studying. Begin the study session with all of the necessary supplies to complete the entire session. Unnecessary breaks to gather additional resources will only serve to prolong or limit the effectiveness of your study session.

Timing

We all function more effectively at specific times of the day. Ideally, study sessions should take place when the mind is alert and attentive. Select a time during the day when you feel you are at your optimal level of functioning. Avoid studying when you are physically tired. Activities such as eating or heavy exercise can lead to decreased attentiveness, and as a result, decrease the effectiveness of your study session. Make sure your emotional state is conducive to learning. If you have had a particularly bad day, avoid studying. Study sessions tend to be unproductive when a candidate is less than 100 percent emotionally.

Frequency and Duration

Studying for short intervals of time has proven to be a more effective learning strategy than studying for long intervals. Specific parameters for frequency and duration are not provided, since they can vary considerably for different learning styles and purposes.

Partnership and Group Recommendations

Many candidates can significantly enhance their preparation for the Physical Therapist Assistant Examination by participating in a study partnership or group. This type of collaboration can offer candidates several distinct benefits:

- Candidates can learn from the information presented by others and as a result reduce their individual study time.

- Candidates can receive assistance from others when remediation is necessary.

- Candidates can assess and modify their individual study plan based on the perceptions and knowledge of others.

Although these arrangements have the potential to be a valuable component of a comprehensive study plan, they need to be structured in a fashion that will allow candidates to be productive. Failure to have adequate structure can result in a study session degenerating into a purely social event. To avoid this potential pitfall, we recommend the following guidelines for all partnerships or groups:

1. Set rules of behavior and a method for staying on task.

2. Set the length and frequency of study sessions, keeping in mind your long-range plan.

3. Set goals that indicate the amount of material to be covered in a specified time period.

4. Establish time during scheduled study sessions to address individual learning needs.

5. Discuss and agree on an agenda for each scheduled study session.

6. Decide on the structure of each study session:

Hierarchical: Someone acts as "teacher" for each session
Participative: Each member acts as facilitator for an area of study
Debate: Exchange of ideas after independent study

7. Attempt to institute a firm schedule for study sessions and emphasize the importance of attendance at each session.

8. Decide on the learning tools the partnership/group will use during each study session.

Candidates should take advantage of available resources, but at the same time recognize there are limits to this type of collaborative approach. It is illegal and unethical to solicit questions from candidates who have taken the examination or to recall and share questions with other candidates after taking the examination. The Federation of State Boards of Physical Therapy will actively prosecute individuals who are engaged in such activities.

Learning Style

The following section offers candidates specific recommendations based on their individual input/processing preferences. Candidates should attempt to utilize this information when participating in a study partnership or group.

Active/Active

Format:
Study sessions should consist of 60-90 minutes of interactive study. The sessions should be designed based on the categories contained within the content outline. Candidates should divide the content outline into smaller, more manageable components.

Many active learners will find it helpful to develop three specific concepts, ideas, or processes to work on for each scheduled study session. After the study session is completed, candidates should make sure they have achieved each established goal. Ample time should be allotted at the end of the study session for a brief review.

Active/Active learners often prefer to divide the workload for the next session. These tasks typically are done independently and usually involve reviewing selected material that will be discussed as part of the next session. This same routine can be repeated with each study session until the actual examination.

Group Composition:

Group members should include learners who are active for input, or processing, or both. There should be a representative sample of left-brain (facts, details) and right-brain (big picture, relationships) dominant candidates.

Frequency:

Since multisensory stimulation is more difficult to achieve alone, it is recommended that study sessions take place as frequently as possible. Daily study sessions would not be considered excessive.

Concerns:

Effective time management is critical, because it can take considerably longer to achieve multisensory stimulation.

Learning Tools:

Color-coding may help in stimulating the visual channel. Discussions, simulations, hands-on practice, and role playing are viable learning activities.

- **Left-brain:** lists, outlines, flow charts
- **Right-brain:** charts, graphs, mind maps

Tips:

Position yourself so that you can observe body language during the study session. Videotapes of sessions may be useful to play back during individual study time to help recreate the study session.

Active/Passive

Format:

Study sessions should be scheduled for a maximum of two hours. The sessions should be designed based on the categories contained within the content outline. Candidates should divide the content outline into smaller, more manageable components.

Many active learners will find it helpful to develop three specific concepts, ideas, or processes to work on for each scheduled study session. After the study session is completed, candidates should make sure they have achieved each established goal.

Ample time should be allotted at the end of the study session for a brief review, and specific tasks should be delegated for the following study session. These tasks typically are done independently and usually involve reviewing selected material that will be discussed as part of the next study session. This same routine can be repeated with each study session until the actual examination.

Although most Active/Passive learners prefer to review information themselves, we recommend that they use a participative format for group work. In this format, each member assumes responsibility for an area of study. Group activity will limit the detailed studying these learners prefer, and provide them with a more comprehensive understanding of the presented material.

Group Composition:
Group members should include learners who are active for input, or processing, or both. There should be a representative sample of left-brain (facts, details) and right-brain (big picture, relationships) dominant candidates.

Frequency:
Two to three times per week is recommended. Candidates may have a desire to reduce the number of sessions; however, they are best served by frequent meetings.

Concerns:
Time management is necessary to maintain concentration and allow for a smooth progression through the content outline.

Learning Tools:
Color-coding may help in stimulating the visual channel. Discussions, simulations, hands-on practice, role playing, and blackboard "teaching" are viable examples.

- **Left-brain:** lists, outlines, flow charts
- **Right-brain:** charts, graphs, mind maps

Tips:
Position yourself so that you can observe body language during the study session. Videotapes of sessions may be useful to play back during individual study time to help recreate the study session.

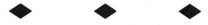

Passive/Active

Format:
Since the majority of studying will take place independently, study sessions should function as an opportunity for candidates to assess their current study plan and benefit from the knowledge of others.

Study sessions should range from two to three hours in length and should focus on large pieces of material. An example of this would be a session at the conclusion of a major section of the content outline.

Group Composition:
Group members should include learners who prefer to study alone and then gather to discuss specific information. Both left and right-brain dominant candidates should be included in the group.

Frequency:
Approximately once per week is recommended. This schedule will allow candidates to cover the necessary material within the established time parameters.

Concerns:
Since the majority of studying has been completed before the review sessions, candidates need to be very careful to include both concepts and applications in their study plan.

Learning Tools:
Blackboard presentations, briefings, debate, occasional simulations.

- **Left-brain:** outlines, lists, flow charts
- **Right-brain:** charts, graphs, mind maps

Tips:
Candidates may have little patience with partners or group members who come to sessions unprepared.

Passive/Passive

Format:
Since the majority of studying will take place independently, study sessions should function as an opportunity for candidates to assess their current study plan and benefit from the knowledge of others.

Study sessions should range from two to three hours in length and should focus on large pieces of material. An example of this would be a session at the conclusion of a major section of the content outline. Since candidates' focus in this category is not on application of material, they should make sure that this area is addressed at each study session.

Group Composition:
Group members should include individuals who prefer to study alone initially. The group should also include members who are application driven.

Frequency:
Approximately once per week is recommended. This schedule will allow candidates to cover the necessary material within the established time parameters.

Concerns:
Time management is necessary to maintain concentration and limit the role of stress.

Learning Tools:
Lectures, blackboard presentations, briefings, observation of simulations, handouts, texts, notes.

- **Left-brain:** outlines, lists, flow charts
- **Right-brain:** charts, graphs, mind maps

Tips:
Passive/Passive learners may become very uncomfortable physically engaging in learning activities before having a chance to review and observe.

Multiple Choice Examinations

Do you believe that Jason Giambi was hitting 450 foot homeruns as a little leaguer or that Serena Williams was consistently hitting blistering passing shots in the second grade? Your answer to these questions is likely to be no. Since history tells us these individuals later accomplished the aforementioned feats, the question becomes, what allowed these individuals to progress to such lofty heights?

The answer probably can best be described in a single word, "practice." Surely individuals like Jason Giambi and Serena Williams were blessed with certain athletic and physical traits which provided them with the opportunity to become successful, but it was their dedication, desire, and determination that allowed them to evolve into superstars in their respective fields.

In physical therapy, there are an abundance of skills that must be learned by the entry level practitioner. Mastery of these skills often requires physical therapist assistants to demonstrate the same type of dedication, desire, and determination exhibited by Jason Giambi and Serena Williams.

Test taking skills are specific skills which allow individuals to utilize the characteristics and format of a selected examination in order to maximize their performance. These skills can be valuable when taking an examination such as the Physical Therapist Assistant Examination. Despite the importance of this topic, very little, if any, academic time is set aside to address test taking skills. The good news is that test taking skills can be learned and that through dedication, desire, and determination, these skills can serve to improve your performance on this important examination.

Since the Physical Therapist Assistant Examination utilizes a multiple choice format, further discussion of test taking skills will be solely concerned with this particular format. Test taking skills can allow candidates to increase their ability to recognize cues within the multiple choice questions. These cues can be utilized to provide valuable information toward identifying the correct response. It has been documented in the literature that recognition of selected cues can lead to improved examination performance.

Individuals who are able to recognize such cues are said to be "test wise." Perhaps this explains, in part, why many students who have prepared adequately for a selected examination often perform poorly. Test taking skills are acquired skills that develop with practice. This unit will present candidates with valuable information on multiple choice examinations and a variety of test taking skills. The unit will also provide candidates with an opportunity to apply the described test taking skills on selected sample examination questions.

Multiple Choice Questions

The Physical Therapist Assistant Examination is a 175 question multiple choice examination that consists of 150 scored items and 25 pretest items. The objective examination consists of multiple choice questions with four potentially correct answers to each question. Candidates are instructed to select the "best answer" to complete each question.

Before we begin to explore selected test taking strategies, we need to identify the various components of a multiple choice question. Multiple choice questions can be dissected into specific identifiable components:

Item: An item refers to an individual multiple choice question and the corresponding potential answers.

Stem: The stem refers to the statement that asks the question.

Options: Options refer to the potential answers to the question asked. One option in each item will be the "best answer," while the others are distracters.

Item:
The Physical Therapist Assistant Examination contains 150 scored items and 25 pretest items. Each item consists of a stem and four options. Items may vary considerably in content and length, but should utilize a consistent format.

Stem:
The stem can take on a variety of forms. Typically, the stem conveys to the reader the necessary information needed to respond correctly to the question. In addition to the necessary information, many times extraneous information is included in the stem. This information, when not recognized by the candidate as unnecessary, often can act as a significant distracter.

The stem commonly can take on the form of a complete sentence, an incomplete sentence, or a fill-in-the-blank. The stem can be expressed in a positive or negative form. A positive form would require a candidate to identify correct information, while a negative form would require a candidate to identify incorrect information. It is important to scrutinize each stem, since a single key word such as "not" or "except" can turn a positive stem into a negative stem. Failure to identify this can lead to the identification of an incorrect answer.

Options:

Options can take on a variety of forms, including a single word, a group of words, an incomplete sentence, a complete sentence, or a group of sentences. The method for analyzing each option does not change, regardless of form.

Question Categorization System

Let's take a few moments to review what we already have learned about the Physical Therapist Assistant Examination. We know that the examination consists of 175 multiple choice questions, each with four possible options. We also know that each question will be representative of one of the three content areas identified in the content outline.

As we introduced in Unit Four, the reporter's formula can be a valuable tool to assist candidates with their preparation for the examination. The reporter's formula utilizes seven specific question words: Who, What, Which, Where, When, How, and Why. By relating each of the question words to the material in the content outline, candidates can effectively review the majority of the information that will be encountered on the Physical Therapist Assistant Examination. By reviewing the information in this manner, candidates gather and store the information in an organized and efficient fashion.

This system can also be utilized to a candidate's advantage when analyzing a multiple choice question. As candidates analyze specific examination questions, they should attempt to categorize each question using the same seven question words. By identifying the correct question word for each of the multiple choice questions, candidates are, in effect, telling the brain where to access the desired information. Since a candidate's study plan was designed in a similar fashion, this process will improve the rate and fluidity of information retrieval. On a timed examination such as the Physical Therapist Assistant Examination, this can be a significant advantage.

It is important for candidates to remember that the purpose of the question categorization system is to assist candidates in understanding the intended meaning of each question. By understanding exactly what each question is asking, candidates can avoid making careless mistakes and improve their examination performance.

Four Levels of Learning & Related Question Types

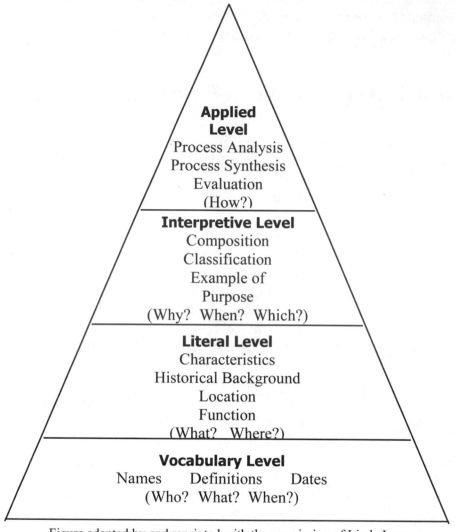

Applied Level
Process Analysis
Process Synthesis
Evaluation
(How?)

Interpretive Level
Composition
Classification
Example of
Purpose
(Why? When? Which?)

Literal Level
Characteristics
Historical Background
Location
Function
(What? Where?)

Vocabulary Level
Names   Definitions   Dates
(Who? What? When?)

Figure adapted by and reprinted with the permission of Linda Lyon.

Of course, we have oversimplified the process, but in your mind you should begin to see how this information can be applied effectively to the Physical Therapist Assistant Examination.

In an attempt to allow candidates to accurately classify examination items, we have divided the seven question words into five separate categories. Selected sample examination questions will be offered to illustrate the use of each category.

Each item in this section will deal with vital signs. Remember, to be classified into a specific category, the exact question word associated with the category does not have to be utilized; rather, think in terms of the problem solving process or the information required to answer the question.

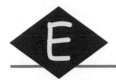

Exercise One

The following exercise contains eleven sample questions for candidates to answer. An answer key is located at the conclusion of the exercise.

Who

This category contains information concerning specific individuals who have made various contributions to the field of physical therapy. It also could include information related to a specific discipline or the responsibilities associated with the discipline.

Sample Question One:
A physical therapist assistant works on an interdisciplinary team in an acute care hospital. One of the patients scheduled to be treated has had severe fluctuations in her blood pressure throughout the night and has been monitored by the nursing staff. Which interdisciplinary team member would be the most appropriate to determine the patient's ability to complete her scheduled rehabilitative session?

1. physical therapist assistant
2. occupational therapist
3. nurse
4. physician

What/Which

This category contains information associated with facts and details. Learning this information typically requires memorization.

What/Which information can be divided into five separate categories:

- Definition
- Characteristics
- Classification
- Composition
- Example

Definition: *meanings of words, terms or procedures*

Sample Question Two:
A physical therapist assistant reviews the medical record of a patient scheduled to be examined in physical therapy. An entry in the medical record indicates the patient has tachycardia. Which description most accurately defines tachycardia?

1. an abnormally fast heart rate
2. an abnormally slow heart rate
3. shortness of breath
4. labored or difficult breathing

Characteristics: *distinguishing traits, qualities, or properties*

Sample Question Three:
A physical therapist assistant records the vital signs of a 42-year-old female at rest. The patient was referred to physical therapy after sustaining a trimalleolar fracture. Which of the following values would not be considered within normal limits?

1. pulse: 82 beats per minute
2. blood pressure: 122/85 mm Hg
3. respiration rate: 20 respirations per minute
4. body temperature: 97.8 °F

Classification: *arranging in, or assigning to, various groups, classes or categories*

Sample Question Four:
A physical therapist assistant measures the blood pressure of a 68-year-old male. The therapist determines the patient's blood pressure is 124/84 mm Hg. This value is best classified as:

1. mild hypotension
2. mild hypertension
3. moderate hypertension
4. within normal limits

Composition: identifying individual elements or arrangements

Sample Question Five:
A physical therapist assistant attempts to calculate a patient's age predicted maximum heart rate. Which of the following is utilized as a component of the age predicted maximum heart rate formula?

1. 180
2. 200
3. 220
4. 240

Example: a representative sample

Sample Question Six:
A physical therapist assistant determines that a patient's blood pressure is elevated when comparing the value obtained during a recent measurement to the patient's normal resting value. Which of the following would tend to increase resting blood pressure?

1. medication
2. anxiety
3. loss of blood
4. decreased cardiac output

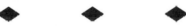

Where

Information in this category usually refers to a location.

Sample Question Seven:
A physical therapist assistant assesses a patient's pulse. In order to accurately assess the patient's apical pulse, the therapist should position the stethoscope:

1. on the chest wall over the apex of the heart
2. over the femoral artery
3. over the carotid artery
4. over the posterior tibial artery

As you can see by answering the Who, What, Which, and Where questions for each of the content areas, there will be very little information that will be omitted from your review. However, you also should recognize that the majority of the material contained within these question words has dealt with fact based information and has not emphasized clinical application. The next series of categories will be more prevalent on the Physical Therapist Assistant Examination. They will deal almost exclusively with clinical application.

How/When

Information in this category involves processes; specifically how to perform tasks step by step and how to analyze what has been done. In some cases, the information follows a sequential timeline (whole-to-part) and sometimes it necessitates drawing together diverse information (part-to-whole) and forming a conclusion.

How/When information can be divided into two categories:

- Process Analysis
- Process Synthesis

Process Analysis: step by step sequencing of information or actions

Sample Question Eight:
A patient sitting in a chair in the physical therapy waiting room suddenly falls to the floor and appears to be unconscious. The physical therapist assistant determines that the patient is not breathing and administers two rescue breaths. The therapist then checks the patient's carotid pulse. If the therapist is able to detect a pulse, he/she should next:

1. begin external chest compressions
2. continue rescue breathing
3. readjust the head tilt and attempt to ventilate
4. determine the pulse rate for 60 seconds

Process Synthesis: *merging of information into "the big picture" and making an informed "action plan"*

Sample Question Nine:
A patient with tetraplegia is two weeks status post cervical spinal fusion. After transferring the patient from the bed to a wheelchair, the patient complains of a severe headache. Upon examination, the patient is found to be diaphoretic and flushed. The patient's blood pressure is recorded as 210/130 mm Hg. These signs and symptoms are most indicative of:

1. autonomic dysreflexia
2. urinary tract infection
3. orthostatic hypotension
4. pulmonary embolus

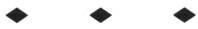

Why

This category typically requires a more advanced level of knowledge than many of the other categories. To answer a Why question successfully, it may be necessary to answer simultaneously What, Which, Where, and/or How information.

Why information can be divided into two categories:

- Cause and Effect
- Function/Use Concepts

Cause and Effect: *relationship between an outcome or state of being and the causative factors*

Sample Question Ten:
A physical therapist assistant attempts to assess the blood pressure of a grossly obese patient. If the bladder of the blood pressure cuff used is too narrow in relation to the circumference of the patient's arm, which of the following would best describe the resultant effect on the patient's measured blood pressure?

1. the value will be erroneously low
2. the value will be erroneously high
3. the value will be reflective of the patient's actual blood pressure
4. the value will not be reflective of the patient's actual blood pressure

Function/Use Concepts: *explanation or rationale for a selected action*

Sample Question Eleven:

A physical therapist assistant establishes a baseline measurement of a patient's vital signs prior to beginning a phase II cardiac rehabilitation program. The primary purpose of conducting the baseline measurement is to:

1. determine the therapeutic measures most appropriate for the patient's rehabilitation program
2. demonstrate objective progress in the patient's rehabilitation program
3. protect the therapist from unnecessary litigation
4. identify significant changes in the values as a result of exercise or other factors

It is possible that many of the examination questions will fall into more than one of the question categories.

Answer Key

1. Answer: 4   Resource: Guide for Professional
                                                        Conduct
   Severe fluctuations in blood pressure can be indicative of a serious medical condition.   The physician is the appropriate professional to assess the patient's changing medical status.

2. Answer: 1   Resource: Minor (p. 39)
   Tachycardia is an abnormally fast heart rate, greater than 100 beats per minute.

3. Answer: 3   Resource: Pierson (p. 59)
   Normal respiration rate in an adult is 12-18 breaths per minute.

4. Answer: 4   Resource: Minor (p. 42)
   124/84 mm Hg is within the accepted blood pressure range for adults.

5. Answer: 3   Resource: Kisner (p. 167)
   Age predicted maximum heart rate is defined as 220 minus age.

6. Answer: 2   Resource: Pierson (p. 59)
   Blood pressure will increase with anxiety and other significant changes in emotional status. Medication may increase or decrease resting blood pressure.

7. Answer: 1   Resource: Pierson (p. 47)
    Auscultation over the apex of the heart using a stethoscope can be used to assess
    the apical pulse.

8. Answer: 2   Resource: American Heart Association
                                                              (p. 75)
    Rescue breathing is indicated for a patient that is not breathing, however does
    have a detectable pulse.

9. Answer: 1   Resource: Pierson (p. 335)
    Autonomic dysreflexia is an exaggerated reflex of the autonomic nervous system.
    It often occurs in individuals with recent spinal cord injuries and is characterized
    by severe hypertension, headache, and sweating.

10. Answer: 2   Resource: Pierson (p. 56)
    A narrow blood pressure cuff will cause the measured value to be high.   The
    width of the bladder should be 40% of the circumference of the midpoint of the
    limb.

11. Answer: 4   Resource: Brannon (p. 250)
    Significant changes in vital signs can only be determined when compared to
    baseline values. This is a fundamental component of all cardiac rehabilitation
    programs.

Task Approach

On the Physical Therapist Assistant Examination there are 175 items that candidates must
answer within a three and one half hour time period. Due to the length of the
examination and the time constraints associated with it, candidates need to approach the
examination in a systematic and organized fashion. Loss of control during the
examination will yield poor results that are not reflective of a candidate's actual
knowledge. We will introduce a four phase process as an example of an approach that
can be used effectively when answering examination questions in a review text or with
slight modification on a computer based test.

Phase I
Carefully read the stem of the first item. Underline key words or groups of words that
offer valuable information. Circle command words that indicate the desired action. If
after reading the stem, you are able to generate an answer to the item, make a mental note
or write the hypothesized answer on scratch paper.

Candidates should then begin to examine each option one at a time. It is important to
read the entire option, since one word often can make a potentially correct answer

incorrect. If the generated answer is consistent with one of the available options, the candidate should give the option strong consideration; however since more than one option can be correct it is imperative to analyze each presented option. If candidates are not able to generate a response, regardless of the reason, they should place an asterisk next to the item number and move to the next item.

Since computer based testing does not allow candidates to mark desired words or phrases, they need to make use of several less direct indicators. These indicators usually take the form of a mental note or a brief written message.

Phase II

Once candidates have completed all of the questions to which they can generate an answer, they should progress to a true/false format. This format allows candidates to have only one potential option in front of them at a time, therefore significantly limiting the distracters.

Candidates should begin by uncovering one of the available options and saying to themselves, "Is it true that ...?" Be sure to substitute the key terms and command words from the stem. Place a "T" or "F" next to the selected option and move to the next option. Continue this pattern until all of the available options have been analyzed. If, after applying this technique, an answer becomes apparent, the candidate should select the answer. If the answer is not apparent, the candidate should move to the next question.

Phase III

By the time a candidate progresses to this phase, the vast majority of the questions on the examination should have been answered. Candidates should return to the beginning of the examination and revisit each remaining question with an asterisk. Candidates again should attempt to generate a response to each of the questions. Likewise, candidates should attempt to analyze unanswered questions by revisiting the true/false format.

Phase IV

At this point there should be very few remaining unanswered questions. Candidates now must utilize deductive reasoning strategies to answer the remaining questions. Deductive reasoning strategies allow candidates to secure points beyond those acquired through direct knowledge of subject matter. Although deductive reasoning strategies are not meant to be used in place of academic knowledge, they have proven to be an effective strategy to improve examination performance.

Deductive reasoning strategies often allow candidates to eliminate one or more of the potential answers. Elimination of any option significantly increases the probability of identifying the correct answer. On the Physical Therapist Assistant Examination, eliminating one option increases the chance of selecting a correct answer from 25% to 33%. Eliminating two options increases the chance of selecting a correct answer to 50%. On the surface this may not seem terribly significant, however on a 175 question test such as the Physical Therapist Assistant Examination this can be the difference between a passing and a failing score. Selected deductive reasoning strategies that can be used effectively on the Physical Therapist Assistant Examination are presented.

- **Absurd Options:** Many times a multiple choice item will include an option that is not consistent with what the stem is asking or with the other options. In many cases, this option can be eliminated. Rapid elimination of specific options will allow candidates to spend additional time analyzing other more viable options.

- **Similar Options:** When two or more options have a similar meaning or express the same fact, they often imply each other's incorrectness. Since candidates are instructed to select the best answer, it would be extremely unlikely that one of two options that are so close in resemblance would be the correct answer. For this reason, candidates can often eliminate both options.

- **Obtainable Information:** There is a great deal of factual material that candidates must sift through when taking the Physical Therapist Assistant Examination. In some instances, the material can provide candidates with valuable information that can assist them in answering other examination questions.

- **Errors in Test Construction:** Since many different individuals are involved in developing the Physical Therapist Assistant Examination, it is difficult to make generalizations about examination construction. Candidates should attempt to answer each question exactly as it is written and avoid the temptation to speculate on the intention of the author.

- **Degree of Qualification:** Particularly in the sciences, there seem to be many exceptions to general rules. Therefore, specific determiners such as "always" or "never" often over qualify an option.

- **Position of the Correct Answer:** Research has demonstrated the tendency for the correct answer in a sequence of alternatives to be at the center of the response distribution. On the Physical Therapist Assistant Examination, the center of the response distribution would correlate to answers 2 and 3.

It is important to remember that deductive reasoning strategies should not be used as a substitute for academic knowledge. Deductive reasoning strategies, when applied indiscriminately or as a substitute for academic knowledge, lead to poor results. Deductive reasoning strategies should be applied only when candidates are unable to identify the correct response using academic knowledge. In these instances, deductive reasoning strategies can be used in combination with academic knowledge to increase the probability of selecting the best answer to a specific examination item.

If after progressing through the four phase process, a candidate still is unable to make an informed decision, he/she should simply attempt to guess at the correct answer. Since there is no penalty associated with guessing on the Physical Therapist Assistant Examination, it is in a candidate's best interest to answer each question.

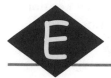

Exercise Two

In this exercise, three sample questions are presented. Candidates should attempt to identify the best answer to each question by utilizing the four phase process. Candidates should also attempt to identify the question type and the specific content area.

The following tables list the possible responses in each category:

Question Category	Content Outline
Who	Tests and Measures (Data Collection)
What/Which	
Where	Intervention
How/When	
Why	Standards of Care

An analysis section immediately follows each of the three sample questions. The analysis section begins by showing the sample question with key terms underlined and command words in bold type. A brief narrative follows, which describes how the four phase process can be applied to the sample question.

An answer key located at the conclusion of the exercise indicates the best answer, question type, and content category for each of the sample questions.

Sample Question One:
A physical therapist assistant instructs a patient with a Foley catheter in ambulation activities. During ambulation the therapist should position the collection bag:

1. above the level of the patient's bladder
2. below the level of the patient's bladder
3. above the level of the patient's heart
4. below the level of the patient's heart

Analysis:

A physical therapist assistant instructs a patient with a <u>Foley catheter in ambulation activities</u>. During ambulation the therapist should **position** <u>the collection bag</u>:

1. above the level of the patient's bladder
2. below the level of the patient's bladder
3. above the level of the patient's heart
4. below the level of the patient's heart

After reading the stem and identifying the pertinent information a candidate should attempt to generate an answer. The candidate then should begin to reveal each of the available options. If a generated answer is consistent with one of the available options, there is a high probability that the answer is correct.

If a candidate was not able to generate an answer, he/she should progress to a true/false format. The candidate will begin this process by creating a true/false statement for each of the available options. The true/false statement for option "1" would be as follows:

> *Is it true that during ambulation the therapist should position the collection bag above the level of the patient's bladder?*

The candidate should answer each question by placing a "T" or "F" next to the corresponding option. He/she should then progress through all of the remaining options in the same manner. Remember, it is possible to have more than one option which satisfactorily answers the question. It is then the candidate's responsibility to select the best answer from the viable options.

Sample Question Two:

A physical therapist assistant monitors a patient's pulse after ambulation activities. The therapist notes that at times the rhythm of the pulse is irregular. When assessing the patient's pulse rate, the therapist should measure the patient's pulse for:

1. 10 seconds
2. 15 seconds
3. 30 seconds
4. 60 seconds

Analysis:
A physical therapist assistant monitors <u>a patient's pulse after ambulation activities</u>.
The therapist notes that <u>at times the rhythm of the pulse is irregular</u>. When <u>assessing
the patient's pulse rate</u>, the therapist should **measure the patient's pulse for:**

1. 10 seconds
2. 15 seconds
3. 30 seconds
4. 60 seconds

After reading the stem and identifying the pertinent information, a candidate will find
that it is difficult to generate a specific answer to the question. A candidate, however,
should immediately begin to focus on the nuances associated with assessing an
irregular pulse.

A candidate should then begin to expose each of the available options. Since in this
specific example all of the options are numerical, it will not be particularly helpful to
apply a true/false format. Instead, a candidate should simply examine the possible
options and attempt to identify the best answer.

In this case, a candidate will need to rely on his/her academic training to answer the
question correctly. It is still, however, important to approach the question in a
systematic fashion in order to avoid making a careless mistake.

Sample Question Three:
A physical therapist assistant completes an isokinetic test on an 18-year-old male
rehabilitating from a medial meniscectomy. The therapist notes that the patient
generates 140 ft/lbs of force using the uninvolved quadriceps at 60 degrees per
second. Assuming a normal ratio of hamstrings to quadriceps strength, which of the
following would be an acceptable hamstrings value at 60 degrees per second?

1. 64 ft/lbs
2. 84 ft/lbs
3. 114 ft/lbs
4. 116 ft/lbs

Analysis:

A physical therapist assistant completes <u>an isokinetic test</u> on an <u>18-year-old male rehabilitating from a medial meniscectomy</u>. The therapist notes that the patient generates <u>140 ft/lbs of force using the uninvolved quadriceps at 60 degrees per second</u>. Assuming <u>a normal ratio of hamstrings to quadriceps strength</u>, which of the following would be **an acceptable hamstrings value** <u>at 60 degrees per second</u>?

1. 64 ft/lbs
2. 84 ft/lbs
3. 114 ft/lbs
4. 116 ft/lbs

For the purpose of discussion, let's assume a candidate has no idea of the normal ratio of quadriceps/hamstrings strength at 60 degrees/second. Lack of specific academic knowledge will result in a candidate not being able to identify the correct answer using a Phase I, Phase II or Phase III approach. However, by applying a Phase IV approach and utilizing deductive reasoning strategies, a candidate can significantly increase his/her chances of identifying the best answer without applying direct academic knowledge.

In this item, the stem asks a candidate to identify a value which would be representative of a normal quadriceps/hamstrings ratio at 60 degrees/second. As with many measurements in physical therapy, precise normal values are difficult to ascertain, and therefore often are expressed in ranges. By applying this knowledge to the examination item, a candidate should be able to eliminate options 3 and 4. Since options 3 and 4 are so close in value they imply each other's incorrectness. Although in this example deductive reasoning strategies were not able to identify the correct answer, they were able to eliminate two of the four possible options. By eliminating the two options, a candidate now has a 50% chance of identifying the best answer, even without utilizing any direct academic or clinical knowledge.

Answer Key

1. Answer: 2   Resource: Pierson (p. 267)
    Question Type: Where
    Content Area: Intervention

    The effect of gravity necessitates the collection bag being positioned below the
    level of the patient's bladder.

2. Answer: 4   Resource: Pierson (p. 52)
    Question Type: Why
    Content Area: Tests and Measures

    Identification of an "irregular" pulse is an indicator to measure for one full
    minute. This method will provide the therapist with the most accurate assessment
    of the patient's actual pulse rate.

3. Answer: 2   Resource: Hamill (p. 236)
    Question Type: Why
    Content Area: Tests and Measures

    A gross estimate of quadriceps:hamstrings ratio is 3:2.

We have attempted to illustrate how the four phase process can be applied to a number of
different sample questions. Although candidates may not always be able to identify the
correct answer using this strategy, when used appropriately, it can serve as a valuable tool
to maximize a candidate's performance on the Physical Therapist Assistant Examination.

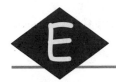

Exercise Three

The following exercise contains ten sample questions for candidates to answer. Resist the urge to approach the questions in a random fashion and instead begin to gain confidence in your ability to answer the questions utilizing the four phase process. An answer key, which is located at the conclusion of the exercise, indicates the best answer, question type, and content category for each of the sample questions.

1. A 16-year-old patient with a complete C5 spinal cord injury is two weeks status post injury. The patient presently tolerates only 30 degrees on the tilt table secondary to orthostatic hypotension. Which transfer would be the most appropriate to utilize when moving the patient from bed to the tilt table?

    1. hydraulic lift
    2. sliding transfer with draw sheet
    3. two person lift
    4. dependent standing pivot transfer

2. Chest percussion and vibration are appropriate bronchial drainage techniques for all of the following except the:

    1. anterior apical segment
    2. lingula
    3. left middle lobe
    4. right middle lobe

3. A patient diagnosed with chondromalacia patellae is referred to physical therapy. During the session, the physical therapist assistant measures the patient's Q angle as 23 degrees bilaterally. Which clinical finding is not typically associated with an increased Q angle?

    1. increased lateral tibial torsion
    2. genu valgum
    3. increased femoral anteversion
    4. patella alta

4. A patient seen twice in physical therapy calls a physical therapist assistant and states that she is no longer interested in therapy and will not return for any additional appointments. The therapist inquires as to the reason for this decision, but the patient refuses to provide any additional information. The therapist's most immediate response should be to:

1. inform the referring physician of the patient's decision
2. document the incident in the medical record
3. call back and ask the patient to reschedule
4. notify the insurance company of the patient's decision

5. A physical therapist assistant designs a treatment program for a patient with a nasogastric tube. Which of the following activities should be avoided when treating the patient?

1. ambulatory distances greater than 100 feet
2. forward bending range of motion exercises of the head and neck
3. static balance activities in sitting
4. shoulder flexion and extension resistive exercises

6. A physical therapist assistant performs passive range of motion to the lower extremities of a patient in the medical intensive care unit. While treating the patient, an alarm on one of the monitoring devices sounds. If the therapist is unfamiliar with the particular piece of monitoring equipment, his most immediate response should be to:

1. contact the patient's referring physician
2. contact a member of the nursing staff
3. attempt to locate a switch to disable the monitoring equipment
4. disregard the alarm and continue with treatment

7. A physical therapist assistant discusses the status of a patient post surgery with a physician. During the discussion the physician cautions the therapist to be alert for any signs or symptoms of pulmonary embolism. Which scenario is most associated with this medical condition?

1. depleted body electrolytes
2. excessive systemic insulin
3. bladder distension
4. thrombus formation

8. A physical therapist assistant assesses wrist radial and ulnar deviation with a goniometer. When measuring radial and ulnar deviation, the therapist should position the axis of the goniometer over the:

    1. capitate
    3. lunate
    3. trapezium
    4. trapezoid

9. Individual health care organizations have the responsibility to safeguard their patients' medical records. Which of the following situations would require prior consent for the use of a patient's medical records?

    1. financial audits
    2. quality assurance
    3. transfer of records to another health care organization
    4. research where anonymity is preserved

10. While ambulating with a transfemoral prosthesis, a patient demonstrates an abducted gait on the prosthetic side. Which of the following is least likely to cause this type of gait deviation?

    1. tightness of the gluteus medius
    2. discomfort on the adductor longus tendon
    3. the medial wall of the prosthesis is too low
    4. the prosthetic limb is too long

Answer Key

1. Answer: 2   Resource: Minor (p. 228)
    Question Type: How/When
    Content Area: Intervention

    A sliding transfer with draw sheet enables the patient to be moved from bed to a
    tilt table without being in an upright position. Since the patient currently only
    tolerates 30 degrees on the tile table the remaining transfer options would not be
    indicated.

2. Answer: 3   Resource: Brannon (p. 43)
    Question Type: What/Which
    Content Area: Intervention

    The left lung does not have a middle lobe.

3. Answer: 4   Resource: Magee (p. 729)
    Question Type: What/Which
    Content Area: Tests and Measures

    A 23 degree Q angle is significantly above the normal value for males or females.
    Patella alta is often associated with a diminished Q angle.

4. Answer: 2   Resource: Kettenbach (p. 31)
    Question Type: How/When
    Content Area: Intervention

    It is necessary for the therapist to document the phone conversation in the medical
    record in a timely fashion.

5. Answer: 2   Resource: Pierson (p. 265)
    Question Type: How/When
    Content Area: Intervention

    A nasogastric tube is a plastic device that is inserted through the nostril and into
    the stomach. Movements of the head and neck can be disruptive.

6. Answer: 2   Resource: Guide for Conduct of the
                                               Physical Therapist Assistant
    Question Type: How/When
    Content Area: Intervention

    Since the therapist is unfamiliar with the monitoring device it is necessary to
    contact another health care professional. The most accessible and logical choice
    would be a member of the nursing staff.

7. Answer: 4   Resource: Hillegass (p. 218)
    Question Type: What/Which
    Content Area: Intervention

    A pulmonary embolism results from a blood clot or thrombus that travels from a
    systemic vein through the right side of the heart into the pulmonary circulation.
    The blood clot or thrombus eventually lodges in the pulmonary artery or one of its
    branches.

8. Answer: 1   Resource: Norkin (p. 88)
    Question Type: Where
    Content Area: Tests and Measures

    When measuring radial and ulnar deviation, the axis of the goniometer is placed
    over the middle of the dorsal aspect of the wrist over the capitate.

9. Answer: 3   Resource: Scott (p. 118)
    Question Type: What/Which
    Content Area: Standards of Care

    Failure to obtain informed consent from a patient prior to releasing medical
    records to another organization can be considered malpractice.

10. Answer: 3   Resource: O'Sullivan (p. 666)
    Question Type: Why
    Content Area: Intervention

    A low medial wall would not cause an abducted gait deviation; a high medial wall
    could be a potential cause.

Recent Developments in Item Construction

There have been a number of changes in item construction on the Physical Therapist Assistant Examination within the past few years, most notably the introduction of paired items and graphically enhanced items. Although representing a relatively small percentage of the total examination, candidates need to be comfortable answering each type of item. Both paired items and graphically enhanced items will be incorporated into the remaining exercises.

Paired Items

Paired items consist of general case information followed by two individual items. Candidates need to use the case information to answer each of the items, although the items themselves remain independent. An example of a paired item is as follows:

The following information should be used to answer questions 1 and 2:

A 65-year-old male diagnosed with chronic obstructive pulmonary disease is referred to physical therapy shortly after being admitted to an acute care hospital. The patient reports that he stopped smoking four weeks ago, however denies any improvement in his exercise tolerance. He is extremely frustrated with his present condition and indicates that even the most basic activities have become extremely difficult.

1. As a component of the treatment regime the physical therapist assistant instructs the patient in pursed-lip breathing. The most appropriate duration of inhalation and exhalation is represented by:

    1. 2 second inhalation; 4 second exhalation
    2. 4 second inhalation; 2 second exhalation
    3. 4 second inhalation; 4 second exhalation
    4. 4 second inhalation; 6 second exhalation

2. The physical therapist assistant uses several objective measures to monitor the patient's response to exercise during the session. Which objective measure would be the most appropriate to avoid hypoxemia?

    1. lung volumes and capacities
    2. blood pressure
    3. oxygen saturation rate
    4. blood glucose level

Graphically Enhanced Items

Graphically enhanced items consist of figures, diagrams, pictures, or other static images that are combined with traditional text in an examination item. An example of a graphically enhanced item is as follows:

The following figure should be used to answer question 3:

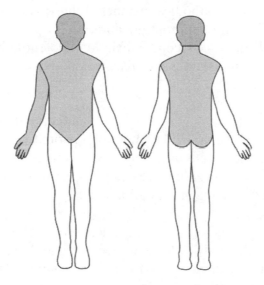

3. A 32-year-old male sustained extensive burns after lighting himself on fire during a suicide attempt. The shaded portion of the body diagrams represent the areas affected by the burns. Using the rule of nines, what percentage of the patient's body was involved?

    1. 40.5%
    2. 44.0%
    3. 49.5%
    4. 54.5%

Answer Key

1. Answer: 4   Resource: Hillegass (p. 736)
    Patients should be instructed to inhale through the nose and exhale through pursed lips in a very slow and methodical manner with exhalation time being greater than inhalation time. The most appropriate duration for pursed-lip breathing is a four second inhalation and a six second exhalation. Potential benefits of pursed-lip breathing include diminished rate of respiration, decreased minute ventilation, and decreased dyspnea.

2. Answer: 3   Resource: Hillegass (p. 665)
    A pulse oximeter can be utilized to monitor a patient's oxygen saturation rate. Hypoxemic states may occur at oxygen saturation levels less than 90%. Modifying the activity level or increasing supplemental oxygen are two methods to address diminished oxygen saturation levels.

3. Answer: 3   Resource: O'Sullivan (p. 852)
    The percentage of the body surface burned in an adult can be calculated using the rule of nines: anterior thorax (18%) + posterior thorax (18%) + head (9%) + anterior arm (4.5%) = 49.5%

Time Constraints

Like many objective examinations, candidates have a specified amount of time to complete the Physical Therapist Assistant Examination. For physical therapist assistants, the available time is three and one half hours. Since the examination consists of 175 questions, candidates will have 72 seconds available to answer each question. This number, although correct when viewing the examination as a whole, can be misleading. There will be many questions that a candidate will be able to answer in much less than 72 seconds, whereas other questions will take somewhat longer. The key to success lies in progressing through the examination in a consistent and predictable manner.

Although 72 seconds per question does not seem like a great deal of time, the majority of candidates will have ample time to complete the examination. Despite this fact, it is important to pay attention to the elapsed time during the examination. It also is important to know your test taking history. Are you typically one of the first, one of the last, or somewhere in the middle of individuals completing an examination? This information is important as you plan your test taking strategy.

In order to make sure your pace is appropriate during practice sessions, we suggest placing a small notation in the margin next to question number 50 and 100. When taking the actual Physical Therapist Assistant Examination, the same objective can be accomplished by writing the question numbers on a piece of paper and placing it next to the computer. These notations should remind candidates to check on the elapsed time at selected intervals throughout the examination. This technique will allow candidates to assess their progress and modify their pace, if needed. Specific guidelines are difficult to determine; however, in general candidates should answer a minimum of 50 questions an hour.

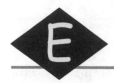

Exercise: Time Management

Candidates will have one hour to complete the following 50 question examination. The allotted time is consistent with the available time per question on the Physical Therapist Assistant Examination. Set a timer for one hour and begin the sample examination. Candidates should use a consistent approach when answering each multiple choice question. After completing the exercise, utilize the answer key located at the conclusion of the exercise to determine the number of questions answered correctly. Record your score for the exercise on the Performance Analysis Summary Sheet located in the Appendix.

1. A physical therapist assistant performs gait training activities with an eight-year-old child who utilizes a reciprocating gait orthosis. Which medical diagnosis is most often associated with the use of this type of orthotic device?

    1. cerebral palsy
    2. Down syndrome
    3. Legg-Calve-Perthes disease
    4. spina bifida

2. A physical therapist assistant reviews the plan of care for a child with a complete L1 spinal cord lesion. The most appropriate functional outcome following a comprehensive rehabilitation program is:

    1. independent ambulation with hip-knee-ankle-foot orthoses and crutches
    2. independent ambulation with knee-ankle-foot orthoses and crutches
    3. independent manual wheelchair mobility
    4. independent power wheelchair mobility

3. A physical therapist assistant employed in an outpatient physical therapy clinic treats a patient with Parkinson's disease. During the session the patient mentions that his physician recently prescribed levodopa. Which symptom of Parkinson's disease would be the most likely to diminish based on the prescribed pharmacological agent?

    1. bradykinesia
    2. sensory disturbances
    3. postural abnormalities
    4. resting tremors

4. A physical therapist assistant attempts to determine the percent body fat of a patient using an objective measure. Which of the following measures would be least appropriate to meet the stated objective?

    1. hydrostatic weighing
    2. skinfold measurements
    3. body mass index
    4. bioimpedance

5. A 29-year-old single mother of three on welfare completes paperwork prior to being examined in physical therapy. The most likely form of third party payment is:

    1. private insurance
    2. Medicare
    3. Medicaid
    4. Workers' compensation

The following information should be used to answer questions 6 and 7:

A physical therapist assistant treats a 72-year-old female recently admitted to an acute care hospital following complications from elective surgery. The patient is moderately obese and has a lengthy medical history including diabetes mellitus. Prior to beginning the treatment session the therapist reviews the patient's medical record.

6. Which measure would provide the most valuable information on the impact of the patient's diabetes on her ability to participate in an exercise program?

    1. arterial blood gas analysis
    2. blood glucose level
    3. oxygen saturation rate
    4. blood pressure

7. The following day the therapist notices that the patient's breath has a very distinctive fruity odor. The patient complains of feeling nauseous and very weak. An entry in the medical record indicates that the patient had diarrhea during the night. This type of scenario is most consistent with:

    1. respiratory acidosis
    2. respiratory alkalosis
    3. metabolic acidosis
    4. metabolic alkalosis

8. A physical therapist assistant treats a 56-year-old male status post transfemoral amputation with a hip flexion contracture. As part of the treatment regime the therapist performs passive stretching exercises to the involved hip. The most appropriate form of passive stretching is:

    1. moderate tension over a prolonged period of time
    2. moderate tension over a brief period of time
    3. maximal tension over a prolonged period of time
    4. maximal tension over a brief period of time

9. A physical therapist assistant treats an infant diagnosed with torticollis with marked lateral flexion of the neck to the right. As part of the infant's plan of care the therapist performs passive stretching activities to improve the patient's range of motion. The most appropriate stretch for the patient is:

    1. lateral flexion to the right and rotation to the right
    2. lateral flexion to the left and rotation to the left
    3. lateral flexion to the right and rotation to the left
    4. lateral flexion to the left and rotation to the right

10. A physical therapist assistant identifies excessive lordosis in a patient during a posture screening. Which of the following findings is most likely associated with this type of spinal curvature?

    1. increased anterior pelvic tilt and lengthened hip extensors
    2. decreased anterior pelvic tilt and shortened hip flexors
    3. increased posterior pelvic tilt and shortened hip extensors
    4. decreased posterior pelvic tilt and lengthened hip flexors

11. A physical therapist assistant interviews a patient referred to physical therapy with a diagnosis of chronic bronchitis. What finding obtained during the patient interview is most closely associated with the patient's medical diagnosis?

    1. patient is a smoker
    2. patient has a sedentary lifestyle
    3. patient has numerous allergies
    4. patient has severe scoliosis

12. A two-year-old child diagnosed with bilateral congenital hip dislocation is referred to physical therapy. The child wears a hip harness designed to stabilize the hip in an attempt to allow the joint capsule to tighten and allow the acetabulum to be properly molded. The most likely position of the hip in the harness is:

    1. hip flexion and abduction
    2. hip flexion and adduction
    3. hip extension and abduction
    4. hip extension and adduction

13. A patient that has difficulty controlling the release and retention of urine uses a urinary catheter. During the treatment session the physical therapist assistant notices that the collection bag is almost completely full. The most appropriate action is to:

    1. continue with the session and periodically monitor the collection bag
    2. disconnect the collection bag during the session
    3. empty the collection bag
    4. contact the patient's nurse and request assistance

14. A physical therapist assistant treats a patient diagnosed with a traumatic brain injury. The patient is classified as level four on the Rancho Los Amigos Level of Cognitive Functioning Scale. Which of the following would be the least appropriate to include in the patient's physical therapy session?

    1. redirection to tasks
    2. random practice, using a variety of tasks
    3. repetition of instructions
    4. ambulation in busy environments

15. A physical therapist assistant reviews the medical record of a 33-year-old male referred to physical therapy with chronic obstructive pulmonary disease. The medical record indicates the patient is 74 inches tall and weighs 184 pounds. The patient's weight is best classified as:

    1. within normal limits
    2. mildly obese
    3. moderately obese
    4. morbidly obese

16. A physical therapist assistant reviews the examination of a patient diagnosed with a cerebellar CVA. The therapist should expect the patient's primary impairment to be:

    1. visual field cuts
    2. decreased balance and coordination
    3. impaired speech
    4. impaired comprehension skills

17. It is essential to maintain a sterile field once it has been established. Which of the following activities would not be in violation of a sterile field?

    1. sneezing while standing in front of a sterile field
    2. reaching across a sterile field
    3. turning your back to the sterile field
    4. allowing a sterile object to touch another sterile object

18. A patient with latissimus dorsi and lower trapezius weakness would have the most difficulty performing which of the following activities?

    1. four-point gait with Lofstrand crutches
    2. three-point gait with a straight cane
    3. swing-through gait with crutches
    4. wheelchair propulsion

19. A physical therapist assistant identifies several inconsistencies between a patient's subjective complaints and objective findings. When completing documentation using a S.O.A.P. note format a discussion of the identified inconsistencies belongs in the:

    1. subjective section
    2. objective section
    3. assessment section
    4. plan section

20. Residual limb wrapping is often a necessary component of a treatment program following lower extremity amputation. Which of the following is not characteristic of a properly applied bandage?

    1. smooth and wrinkle free
    2. emphasizes angular turns
    3. provides pressure distally
    4. encourages proximal joint flexion

21. A physical therapist assistant determines that a patient rehabilitating from ankle surgery has consistent difficulty with functional activities that emphasize the frontal plane. Which of the following activities would be the most difficult for the patient?

    1. anterior lunge
    2. 6 inch lateral step down
    3. 6 inch posterior step up
    4. 8 inch posterior step down

The following figure or diagram should be used to answer question 22:

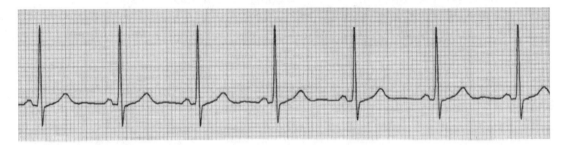

22. A patient is required to have an electrocardiogram as part of a physical examination. A rhythm strip from the electrocardiogram while the patient was at rest is displayed above. Assuming the patient's heart rate was determined to be 70 beats per minute, the heart rate is most representative of:

    1. sinus bradycardia
    2. normal sinus rhythm
    3. sinus arrhythmia
    4. sinus tachycardia

23. A physical therapist assistant completes ambulation activities with a patient rehabilitating from a total hip replacement. Later while documenting in the medical record, the therapist realizes she has exceeded the patient's prescribed weight bearing status. The most immediate therapist action is to:

    1. disregard the incident
    2. discuss the situation with the director of rehabilitation
    3. inform the orthopedic surgeon of the incident
    4. complete an incident report

24. A patient with chronic venous insufficiency presents with significant edema in both lower extremities. Which treatment option would be the most appropriate for the initial visit?

    1. intermittent compression and patient education
    2. custom fitted stockings
    3. intermittent compression and warm whirlpool
    4. instruction in a lower extremity exercise program

25. A physical therapist assistant monitors a patient's respiration rate during exercise. Which of the following would be considered a normal response?

    1. the respiration rate declines during exercise before the intensity of exercise declines
    2. the respiration rate does not increase during exercise
    3. the rhythm of the respiration pattern becomes irregular during exercise
    4. the respiration rate decreases as the intensity of the exercise plateaus

26. A physical therapist assistant observes the skin of a 42-year-old patient diagnosed with multiple sclerosis. The therapist identifies a pressure ulcer approximately two centimeters in diameter near the patent's left ischial tuberosity. The ulcer looks like an abrasion and appears to involve the entire epidermis. The ulcer is best classified as:

    1. stage I
    2. stage II
    3. stage III
    4. stage IV

27. A physical therapist assistant treats a patient diagnosed with suspected arterial occlusive disease. The therapist identifies a number of findings consistent with the diagnosis including absent femoral pulse, dependent rubor, and intermittent claudication in the buttocks, hamstrings, and calf muscles. The most likely site of occlusion is the:

    1. iliac artery
    2 femoral artery
    3. popliteal artery
    4. tibial artery

28. A patient rehabilitating from a fractured humerus develops a resultant musculocutaneous nerve lesion. Which objective finding is most indicative of musculocutaneous nerve involvement?

    1. weakness of shoulder medial rotation
    2. sensory loss in the lateral forearm
    3. winging of the inferior angle of the scapula
    4. loss of contour in the shoulder due to deltoid paralysis

29. An administrator in a rehabilitation hospital presents an inservice on legal and ethical issues for health care practitioners. During the inservice the administrator reviews several types of law that affect the health care system. Which type of law is based on court judgments, decisions, and decrees?

    1. constitutional law
    2. statutory law
    3. common law
    4. administrative law

30. A patient in an acute care hospital attempts to get out of bed in preparation for ambulation activities. The patient has not been able to ambulate since being admitted to the hospital four weeks ago. The most immediate physical therapist assistant action is to:

    1. disconnect the patient's intravenous line
    2. provide a straight cane for ambulation activities
    3. have the patient sit on the edge of the bed with his feet on the floor
    4. instruct family members in various transfer techniques

31. A physical therapist assistant performs daily goniometric measurements on a patient status post total knee arthroplasty. To ensure the most reliable goniometric measurement, the therapist should:

    1. utilize the same goniometer for each measurement
    2. accurately identify appropriate bony landmarks
    3. perform goniometric measurements at the same time each day
    4. provide the patient with concise and explicit verbal instructions

32. A patient rehabilitating from a CVA exhibits signs and symptoms of depression. Which of the following is not representative of a patient with depression?

    1. the patient develops unrealistic rehabilitation goals
    2. the patient exhibits decreased participation in physical therapy
    3. the patient expresses feelings of worthlessness
    4. the patient exhibits periods of agitation and loss of energy

33. A physical therapist assistant treats a patient referred to physical therapy with a cervical strain. During the session the therapist begins to suspect there may be a lesion interfering with neural conduction. Which resisted test would supply the therapist with information on the C4 myotome?

    1. elbow extension
    2. shoulder abduction
    3. shoulder shrug
    4. elbow flexion

34. A 72-year-old male status post CVA is referred to physical therapy. The patient is able to ambulate independently and has good upper extremity strength, however is unable to communicate through verbal or written means. This type of deficit is best termed:

    1. apraxia
    2. aphasia
    3. aphonia
    4. aplasia

35. As part of a quality assurance program, a physical therapy department embarks on an outcome assessment study. When working with outcome assessment the most critical period of time is:

    1. at the conclusion of a selected treatment session
    2. at the conclusion of care in relation to the goals of treatment
    3. at the conclusion of a 14 day period
    4. after a scheduled physician visit

36. A patient is diagnosed with a bacterial infection shortly after being admitted to the hospital. Which of the following laboratory tests would you expect to be most affected based on the patient's diagnosis?

    1. platelet count
    2. hemoglobin
    3. hematocrit
    4. white blood cell count

The following information should be used to answer questions 37 and 38:

A physical therapist assistant suspects the presence of a deep vein thrombosis in a 52-year-old female status post surgery. The therapist became concerned after the patient complained of pain and tenderness in the calf and a physical examination revealed increased topical warmth and distal swelling. Based on the information, the therapist decides to contact the referring physician.

37. Which test or measure would be the most appropriate to confirm the presence of a deep vein thrombosis?

    1. Doppler ultrasonography
    2. Homans' sign
    3. prothrombin time
    4. complete blood count

38. After confirming the presence of deep vein thrombosis in the patient's calf, the physician places the patient on heparin. Assuming the absence of additional complications, how long until the patient is able to return to her normal activity level without restrictions?

    1. 2-5 days
    2. 1-3 weeks
    3. 4-8 weeks
    4. 3 months

39. A patient diagnosed with chronic venous insufficiency is referred to physical therapy. The patient's plan of care is designed to increase venous return and reduce edema. Which of the following would not be part of the expected plan of care?

    1. manual massage of the extremities in a proximal to distal direction
    2. use of an intermittent compression pump
    3. avoid prolonged periods of static standing and sitting with legs dependent
    4. elevation of the foot of the bed during rest

40. A 65-year-old female rehabilitating from a motor vehicle accident is referred to therapy for treatment of lymphedema. Which of the following would not be part of the expected plan of care?

    1. application of local heat
    2. isometric and isotonic pumping exercises of the distal muscles
    3. elevation of the extremity above the level of the heart
    4. intermittent mechanical compression

41. A physical therapist assistant treats a 55-year-old male whose subjective complaints include asymmetric pain in the knees and hips. The patient describes the intensity of the pain in proportion to the amount of daily activity. The patient indicates he has been employed as a roofer for the past 20 years. Which disease category is most consistent with this case?

    1. systemic lupus erythematosus
    2. osteoarthritis
    3. rheumatoid arthritis
    4. gout

42. A patient diagnosed with a grade I anterior talofibular ligament sprain is referred to physical therapy. The best indicator of the patient's expected functional status following rehabilitation would be based on:

    1. the patient's previous functional status
    2. the number of physical therapy visits
    3. the quality of the physical therapy services
    4. the patient's willingness to complete a home exercise program

43. A physical therapist assistant instructs a patient with a lower extremity amputation to wrap her residual limb. Which of the following would be the least acceptable method of securing the bandages?

    1. clips
    2. safety pins
    3. tape
    4. velcro

44. A physical therapist assistant reviews a research study that examines the effect of age on range of motion of the spine and extremities. When comparing infants to adults, which of the following statements would be incorrect?

    1. infants have more hip flexion range of motion than adults
    2. infants have more knee extension range of motion than adults
    3. infants have more ankle dorsiflexion range of motion than adults
    4. infants have more hip lateral rotation range of motion than adults

45. A patient rehabilitating from congestive heart failure exercises in physical therapy. During the session the patient begins to complain of pain. The most appropriate physical therapist assistant action is to:

    1. notify the nursing staff to administer pain medication
    2. contact the referring physician
    3. discontinue the treatment session
    4. ask the patient to describe the location and severity of the pain

46. A physical therapist assistant prepares to treat a patient who is one week status post CVA. When observing the patient lying in bed, the therapist notes that the patient's calf and foot are edematous. The patient reports that the area is somewhat painful. The therapist should:

    1. discontinue treatment and hope the patient's leg is better tomorrow
    2. consider ordering compression stockings for the patient
    3. continue with treatment and disregard the patient's condition
    4. inform the physician of the situation and discontinue treatment

47. A physical therapist assistant discontinues an exercise session after a patient exhibits signs and symptoms of acute angina. The most effective formal method to communicate this information to the supervising physical therapist is through:

1. direct verbal contact
2. the medical record
3. the patient's nurse
4. the referring physician

48. A physical therapist assistant strongly suspects a patient is intoxicated after arriving for his treatment session. When asked if he has been drinking, the patient indicates he consumed six or seven alcoholic beverages before driving to therapy. The therapist's most appropriate action is to:

1. continue to treat the patient, assuming he can remain inoffensive to other patients
2. modify the patient's present treatment program to minimize the effects of alcohol
3. contact a member of the patient's family to take the patient home
4. instruct the patient to leave the clinic

49. A physical therapist assistant covering for another therapist on vacation treats a patient with C5-C6 tetraplegia. During the treatment session the patient's spouse asks a question regarding the patient's ability to transfer independently following rehabilitation. The most appropriate therapist response is to:

1. refer the spouse to the director of rehabilitation
2. refer the spouse to the patient's primary physician
3. refer the spouse to the patient's primary nurse
4. answer the spouse's question

50. A physical therapist assistant reviews the medical record of a patient recently admitted to the hospital. A specific entry in the medical record contains the word hyperglycemic. This word can best be defined as:

1. excessive bleeding
2. excessive amounts of sugar in the blood
3. excessive carbon dioxide in the blood
4. excessive numbers of red blood cells

Answer Key

1. Answer: 4   Resource: Campbell - Decision Making
                                                       (p. 212)
   A reciprocating gait orthosis is a type of hip-knee-ankle orthosis that incorporates
   a cable connecting the two hip joint mechanisms. The orthosis is most commonly
   utilized with children diagnosed with spina bifida.

2. Answer: 1   Resource: Long (p. 69)
   A child with a complete L1 spinal cord lesion would possess full upper extremity
   and trunk function, however would not possess intact lower extremity
   musculature. As a result, the child would require hip-knee-ankle-foot orthoses
   and crutches for independent ambulation.

3. Answer: 1   Resource: Ciccone (p. 123)
   Levodopa can dramatically improve bradykinesia and rigidity in patients with
   Parkinson's disease. Approximately 80% of patients taking levodopa experience
   various forms of dyskinesia including tremors, dystonia, and ballismus.

4. Answer: 3   Resource: American College of Sports
                                                       Medicine (p. 63)
   Body mass index (BMI) is used to assess weight relative to height, however it is
   not used to assess percent body fat since it does not consider fat-free density and
   skeletal mass.

5. Answer: 3   Resource: Sultz (p. 245)
   Medicaid is a program that provides medical and health related services to
   qualifying individuals and families with low income and resources. Medicaid is a
   joint venture between the Federal and State governments. Medicaid federal
   guidelines require states to offer a mandatory core of basic medical services
   including inpatient and outpatient hospital services, physician services, diagnostic
   services, nursing home care, home health care, preventive care, health screening
   services, and family planning services.

6. Answer: 2   Resource: Goodman – Pathology
                                                       (p. 1182)
   Blood glucose level is used as an indicator of carbohydrate metabolism and is
   commonly assessed in patients with diabetes. Normal blood glucose values range
   from 80-120 mg/dL.

7. Answer: 3   Resource: Goodman – Pathology
                                                        (p. 116)
Metabolic acidosis usually results from an excess accumulation of acids in the
blood. Patients with uncontrolled diabetes may be particularly susceptible to
ketoacidosis which is characterized by a fruity breath odor resulting from a build
up of acids. The condition warrants immediate medical intervention.

8. Answer: 1   Resource: Kisner (p. 184)
Moderate tension over a prolonged period of time would be the most appropriate
form of stretching for the hip flexors. In addition, this type of stretch will be more
readily tolerated by the patient.

9. Answer: 4   Resource: Long (p. 190)
Torticollis is a condition caused by a contracture of the sternocleidomastoid
muscle. The condition is characterized by lateral flexion of the head toward the
affected side and rotation toward the unaffected side.   Stretching activities should
be performed in the opposite direction.

10. Answer: 1   Resource: Kendall (p. 80)
Lordosis refers to an abnormal anterior convexity of the spine. Lordosis most
commonly results in shortened hip flexors and lengthened hip extensors.

11. Answer: 1   Resource: Hillegass (p. 274)
Chronic bronchitis is characterized by increased mucus secretion sufficient to
produce a productive cough for at least three months during two consecutive
years. Cigarette smoking is the most commonly cited causal factor in the
development of chronic bronchitis.

12. Answer: 1   Resource: Goodman - Pathology
                                                        (p. 596)
Hip flexion and abduction provide the optimal position for tightening of the joint
capsule and molding of the acetabulum. The most common type of hip harness
for children with congenital hip dysplasia is the Pavlick harness.

13. Answer: 4   Resource: Pierson (p. 267)
Failure to allow for adequate flow of urine into a collection bag can lead to
serious medical complications. It is also often necessary for the nusing staff to
inspect and measure the amount of urine collected.

14. Answer: 4   Resource: O'Sullivan (p. 800)
Patients that are confused-agitated are often over stimulated by busy
environments.

15. Answer: 1   Resource: Bickley (p. 83)
The question does not specify the patient's frame size (small, medium, large), however a weight of 184 pounds for a male that is 6 feet two inches should be considered within normal limits.

16. Answer: 2   Resource: O'Sullivan (p. 159)
Characteristics of cerebellar lesions include diminished coordination, decreased muscle tone, and impaired balance.

17. Answer: 4   Resource: Pierson (p. 293)
Sterile objects that touch each other are still considered sterile.

18. Answer: 3   Resource: Pierson (p. 299)
A swing-through gait pattern with crutches requires significant upper extremity strength and scapular stability. The gait pattern is often used with patients who have bilateral lower extremity weakness or paralysis.

19. Answer: 3   Resource: Kettenbach (p. 110)
The assessment section of a S.O.A.P. note provides a platform for a therapist to express his/her professional judgment.

20. Answer: 4   Resource: Ellis (p. 15)
Encouraging proximal joint flexion can lead to contractures.

21. Answer: 2   Resource: Norkin (p. 5)
The frontal plane divides the body into front and back halves. Movements in the frontal plane occur as side to side movements such as abduction or adduction. Rotary motion in the frontal plane occurs around an anterior-posterior axis.

22. Answer: 2   Resource: Irwin (p. 55)
A normal sinus rhythm has an impulse that originates from the SA node and follows the normal conduction pathways during depolarization. Resting heart rates typically range from 60 to 100 beats per minute.

23. Answer: 4   Resource: Scott (p. 69)
An incident report should be completed which will serve to provide details of the event in question.

24. Answer: 1   Resource: Kisner (p. 718)
The primary goal of treatment is to increase venous return and reduce edema. Intermittent compression will assist with this goal and patient education will be directed toward decreasing dependent edema.

25. Answer: 4   Resource: Pierson (p. 61)
As the intensity of exercise plateaus, a patient will accommodate to the level of exercise and his/her respiration rate will tend to decrease.

26. Answer: 2   Resource: Goodman – Pathology
                                                        (p. 308)
A stage II ulcer is characterized by partial-thickness skin loss involving the epidermis and/or dermis. The ulcer is usually superficial and may present as an abrasion, blister, or crater.

27. Answer: 1   Resource: Goodman – Pathology
                                                        (p. 452)
Occlusive disease of the iliac artery would likely result in significant findings throughout the lower extremities. Intermittent claudication extending into the buttock area and an absent femoral pulse combine to make the iliac artery the most probable site for occlusion.

28. Answer: 2   Resource: Rothstein (p. 316)
The musculocutaneous nerve (C5, C6, C7) innervates the biceps brachii, coracobrachialis, and the majority of the brachialis. The nerve supplies cutaneous innervation to the lateral forearm via the lateral cutaneous nerve. The musculocutaneous nerve is often injured in fractures or dislocations of the humerus.

29. Answer: 3   Resource: Scott (p. 5)
Common law develops over time based on judicial decisions. It is also referred to as judge-made case law.

30. Answer: 3   Resource: Goodman-Pathology (p. 296)
Since the patient has been in bed a significant amount of time without ambulating it is advisable to assist him/her to a standing position in a gradual fashion. This will help to avoid the patient feeling light headed, dizzy, or exhibiting signs of postural hypotension.

31. Answer: 2   Resource: Norkin (p. 35)
Although each of the options has an influence on the reliability of goniometric measurements, identifying the appropriate bony landmarks is fundamental to any goniometric measurement.

32. Answer: 1   Resource: Bickley (p. 599)
Depression is defined as a morbid sadness, dejection, or melancholy; distinguished from grief, which is realistic and proportionate to a personal loss.

33. Answer: 3   Resource: Kendall (p. 282)
The trapezius is innervated by the spinal portion of cranial nerve XI and ventral ramus of C2, C3, and C4. The upper trapezius assists with the ability to approximate the acromion and occiput.

34. Answer: 2   Resource: Anderson (p. 122)
Aphasia is defined as the loss of power of expression by speech, writing, or signs due to disease or injury of the brain center.

35. Answer: 2   Resource: Walter (p. 244)
Outcome assessment studies tend to compare a patient's status at the time of discharge in relation to the expected goals of treatment.

36. Answer: 4   Resource: Goodman-Differential
                                                 Diagnosis (p. 185)
Lymphocytes, monocytes, and granulocytes are types of white blood cells encountered with infection.

37. Answer: 1   Resource: Goodman – Pathology
                                                 (p. 458)
Doppler ultrasonography is the most effective method to determine the presence of deep vein thrombosis (DVT). Homans' sign is still commonly utilized, however research indicates that the test may be positive in only 30% of documented cases of DVT.

38. Answer: 2   Resource: Goodman – Pathology
                                                 (p. 459)
Patients that are treated with anticoagulation medication following the identification of a deep vein thrombosis in the calf can usually return to their previous activity level in 1-3 weeks. Patients with a deep vein thrombosis in the thigh or pelvic region may require six weeks or longer.

39. Answer: 1   Resource: Kisner (p. 718)
Massage techniques utilized on a patient with chronic venous insufficiency should be in a distal to proximal direction.

40. Answer: 1   Resource: Kisner (p. 721)
Application of local heat will place an increased demand on the lymphatic system and should therefore be avoided.

41. Answer: 2   Resource: Pauls (p. 82)
Osteoarthritis is a chronic degenerative disorder that leads to the breakdown of the articular cartilage of synovial joints. Joints most commonly affected are the weight bearing joints. Pain is typically worse with activity and morning stiffness is often present.

42. Answer: 1   Resource: Hertling (p. 423)
A grade I ligament sprain is a relatively minor injury that is often resolved in 2-3 weeks. As a result, the patient's previous functional status should serve as an ideal predictor of functional status following rehabilitation.

43. Answer: 1   Resource: O'Sullivan (p. 630)
Clips often provide poor anchors and can cut the skin. Safety pins are also of questionable value, however are not as dangerous as clips.

44. Answer: 2   Resource: Campbell – Physical Therapy
                                                          (p. 133)
Studies have shown that newborns and infants present with limited hip and knee extension when compared to adults.

45. Answer: 4   Resource: Magee (p. 3)
Although a subjective report of pain is relevant information, additional information must be gathered prior to determining its significance.

46. Answer: 4   Resource: Paz (p. 376)
The patient's signs and symptoms are consistent with the presence of a deep venous thrombosis. Referral for additional examination is necessary.

47. Answer: 2   Resource: Hickock (p. 105)
Formal communication should be part of the permanent or lasting record. Verbal communication is not a formal method of communication.

48. Answer: 3   Resource: Guide for Conduct of the
                                                          Physical Therapist Assistant
The patient is likely to be intoxicated if he has consumed six or seven beers. Contacting a member of the family will prevent the possibility of the patient attempting to drive.

49. Answer: 2   Resource: Guide for Conduct of the
                                                          Physical Therapist Assistant
The question asked by the spouse falls outside the assistant's scope of practice, particularly since the assistant is providing coverage for another therapist. The most appropriate response would be to encourage the spouse to consult with the physician.

50. Answer: 2   Resource: Goodman-Pathology (p. 251)
Hyperglycemia often occurs as a complication of diabetes mellitus. Symptoms of hyperglycemia include thirst, polyuria, lethargy, and confusion.

This activity should have provided candidates with a basic understanding of the time available to answer a selected number of questions. Candidates should, however, recognize that taking a 50 question examination in one hour is much different than taking the actual Physical Therapist Assistant Examination. Issues such as the environment, concentration, and endurance, which for most candidates are not as relevant when taking a 50 question examination, can be very relevant when candidates are subjected to the actual examination.

The most effective way to determine if the time constraints of the Physical Therapist Assistant Examination will affect you is to practice taking 150 question sample examinations. This activity will not only reduce your anxiety level about the time constraints, but will also allow you to make changes in your pace, if necessary, prior to the actual examination.

Unit Eight contains a 150 question sample examination. Additional information on review books and computer software designed for the Physical Therapist Assistant Examination is located at the conclusion of the text.

Content Outline

Perhaps the most valuable piece of information a candidate can utilize when preparing for the Physical Therapist Assistant Examination is the content outline. The content outline provides a detailed analysis of each of the three content areas of the Physical Therapist Assistant Examination. A thorough understanding of each of the content areas and the corresponding subtopics will streamline a candidate's preparation. Less time will be spent covering topics that are not clinically relevant to the actual examination and as a result, more time will be available for reviewing and relearning.

The chart below illustrates the three content areas of the Physical Therapist Assistant Examination and the percentage of examination items in each content area.

Physical Therapist Assistant Examination Content Outline

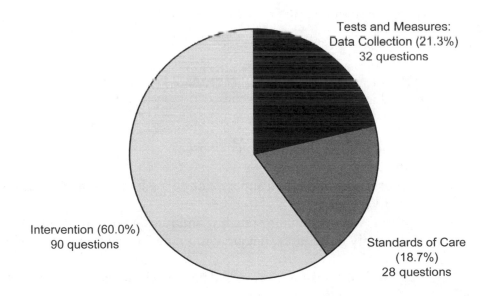

Tests and Measures: Data Collection (21.3%) 32 questions

Standards of Care (18.7%) 28 questions

Intervention (60.0%) 90 questions

Content Outline

Federation of State Boards of Physical Therapy

Physical Therapist Assistant Examination

I. **Tests and Measures (Data Collection)**

   Tests and Measures Group I
   1. Strength, ROM, Posture, Body Structures
   2. Cognition, Reflex and Sensory Integrity

   Tests and Measures Group II
   1. Cardiovascular/pulmonary System – endurance, circulation, physiological status, ventilation, respiration tests
   2. Integumentary System – observe patient skin status; observe and measure patient wounds (e.g. size, depth)
   3. Functional Status – assistive and adaptive devices, gait, balance, pain, body mechanics

II. **Intervention**

   Non-procedural Interventions
   1. Coordination of care
   2. Interpersonal communication
   3. Documentation
   4. Patient/family/client-related instructions

   Procedural Interventions
   Group I: Exercise and manual therapy

   Group II: Transfer and functional activities, gait training, assistive and adaptive devices, and modification of the environment

   Group III: Physical agents and modalities

   Group IV: Airway clearance techniques, wound care, promoting health and wellness, and intervention effectiveness

III. **Standards of Care**

   A. Patient confidentiality, autonomy, and consent
   B. Work Parameters
      1. Work under the direction and supervision of a PT in an ethical, legal, safe, and effective manner
      2. Knowing and working within state law and rules governing physical therapy
      3. Performing only those tasks that are within the PTAs knowledge and skill level
      4. Utilizing clinical decision making in data collection and interventions
   C. Body mechanics/positioning/draping
   D. Safety, CPR, emergency care, first aid
   E. Standard precautions

The actual number of questions in each content area for the 150 question Physical Therapist Assistant Examination can be determined based on the given percentage of examination items. The following table identifies the number of questions in each of the three content areas on the Physical Therapist Assistant Examination.

Content Areas	Number of Questions
Tests and Measures (Data Collection)	32
Intervention	90
Standards of Care	28
	Total = 150

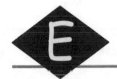

Exercise: Content Outline Analysis

The following exercise will explore the content outline in greater detail. A general statement regarding the subject matter in each subtopic is presented along with an outline of associated information. The information is obtained from the current content outline published by the Federation of State Boards of Physical Therapy.

Ten sample questions will be presented for candidates to answer in each subtopic. Candidates should recognize that these questions represent only a small fraction of the potential questions that could appear on the actual examination. Additional sample questions for each of the subtopics will appear in the sample examination contained in Unit Eight. Candidates should use this exercise not only to become familiar with the content outline, but also to refine their test taking skills.

Candidates will have a maximum of one hour and 36 minutes to complete the 80 questions. Attempt to identify the best answer for each of the questions. After completing the exercise, utilize the answer key located at the conclusion of the exercise to determine the number of questions answered correctly. Record your score for the exercise on the Performance Analysis Summary Sheet located in the Appendix.

Physical Therapist Assistant Examination
Content Outline Analysis

I. *Tests and Measures (Data Collection)*

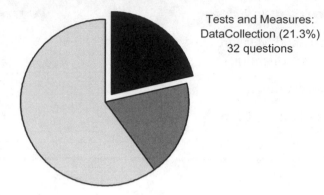

Tests and Measures:
DataCollection (21.3%)
32 questions

Examination	Number of Questions
Test and Measures Group I	17
Test and Measures Group II	15
	Total = 32

Test and Measures: Group I

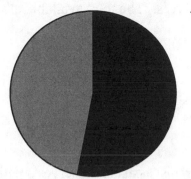

Tests and Measures Group I
17 questions

Group I:

Strength, ROM, Posture, Body Structures, Prosthetic & Orthotic Devices
    Anthropometric characteristics – measure extremity, girth, and length
    Posture – observe patient posture
    Range of Motion/muscle length – measure patient range of motion
    Muscle performance – perform manual muscle testing techniques

Cognition, Nerve, Reflex and Sensory Integrity, Neurodevelopment
    Arousal, attention, and cognition – check patient cognitive status
    Reflex integrity – check patient muscle tone
    Sensory integrity – test patient sensation, proprioception, and kinesthesia

Sample Questions

1. A physical therapist assistant passively moves a patient's upper extremity through a selected range of motion while the patient's eyes are closed. The patient is then asked to verbally describe the direction and range of movement of the upper extremity. This technique can be used to assess:

    1. barognosis
    2. graphesthesia
    3. kinesthesia
    4. stereognosis

2. A physical therapist assistant completes an upper extremity goniometric measurement. The therapist records right active elbow range of motion as 15 - 0 - 150 degrees. The total available elbow range of motion for this patient is:

   1. 135 degrees
   2. 150 degrees
   3. 165 degrees
   4. 180 degrees

3. A physical therapist assistant observes a patient with unilateral lower extremity weakness complete an exercise program. As the patient performs hip flexion in supine the therapist helps the patient complete the full range of motion. This would best be described as:

   1. active exercise
   2. passive exercise
   3. resistive exercise
   4. active-assistive exercise

4. A patient recently involved in a motor vehicle accident is referred to physical therapy after being diagnosed with a cervical strain. During the session the physical therapist assistant palpates the anterior aspect of the neck. Which of the following bony structures is most superior?

   1. thyroid cartilage
   2. first cricoid ring
   3. hyoid bone
   4. C5 vertebral body

5. A physical therapist assistant classifies end-feel at a selected joint as firm after completing a passive range of motion test. A firm end-feel is most indicative of:

   1. capsular or ligamentous stretching
   2. bone contacting bone
   3. soft tissue approximation
   4. joint effusion

6. A physical therapist assistant treats a 40-year-old female referred to physical therapy after spraining her ankle playing volleyball. During the session the patient exhibits extreme tenderness to palpation over the sinus tarsi. What ligament is most often associated with tenderness in this area?

    1. anterior talofibular
    2. calcaneofibular
    3. deltoid
    4. posterior talofibular

7. A physical therapist assistant attempts to determine the end-feel associated with knee flexion. Assuming a normal end-feel, which of the following classifications is most appropriate?

    1. soft
    2. firm
    3. hard
    4. empty

8. A physical therapist assistant measures a patient's subtalar range of motion. When goniometrically assessing subtalar range of motion, the moving arm of the goniometer should be positioned over the:

    1. posterior midline of the calcaneus
    2. anterior aspect of the ankle midway between the malleoli
    3. over the posterior aspect of the ankle between the malleoli
    4. anterior midline of the second metatarsal

9. A physical therapist assistant assesses the sensation of a patient with incomplete T7-T8 paraplegia using a piece of cotton. The therapist applies the cotton in a random fashion and asks the patient to indicate when he feels the stimulus. This method of sensory testing is used to assess:

    1. kinesthesia
    2. light touch
    3. proprioception
    4. superficial pain

10. A physical therapist assistant records a manual muscle test grade of poor for right hip adduction. The most appropriate patient position to conduct the test would be:

   1. supine
   2. prone
   3. right sidelying
   4. left sidelying

Test and Measures: Group II

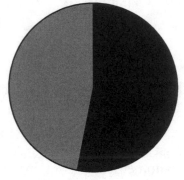

Tests and Measures Group II
15 questions

Group II:

Cardiovascular/pulmonary System
   Aerobic capacity/endurance
   Circulation – utilize appropriate circulation tests; use appropriate tests to measure patient physiological status (e.g., vital signs, blood pressure, heart rate)
   Ventilation and respiration/gas exchange – utilize appropriate ventilation, respiration tests

Integumentary System
   Integumentary integrity – observe patient skin status; observe and measure patient wounds (e.g., size, depth)

Functional Status and Community Integration
   Assistive and adaptive devices – identify need and measure for assistive devices (canes, wheelchairs, etc.)
   Gait, locomotion, and balance – observe patient gait, test patient balance
   Pain – check patient pain
   Ergonomics and body mechanics – observe body mechanics

Sample Questions

11. A physical therapist assistant observes a burn on the dorsal surface of a patient's arm. The therapist notes that the wound appears to involve the epidermis and most of the dermis. The wound area is mottled red with a number of blisters. The physical therapist assistant informs the patient that healing should take place in less than three weeks. This description is most indicative of a:

    1. superficial burn
    2. superficial partial-thickness burn
    3. deep partial-thickness burn
    4. full-thickness burn

12. A physical therapist assistant treats a patient who complains of occasional difficulty maintaining her balance when walking and frequent episodes of vertigo. The most likely cause of the patient's difficulty is a disorder of the:

    1. visual system
    2. proprioceptive system
    3. auditory system
    4. vestibular system

13. A physical therapist assistant attempts to obtain information on a patient's endurance level while exercising on a treadmill. Which of the following measurement methods would provide the therapist with an objective measure of endurance?

    1. facial color
    2. facial expression
    3. rating on a perceived exertion scale
    4. respiratory rate

14. A physical therapist assistant monitors a 6 foot 3 inch, 275 pound male's blood pressure using the brachial artery. Which of the following is the most important factor when selecting an appropriate size blood pressure cuff?

    1. patient age
    2. percent body fat
    3. somatotype
    4. extremity circumference

15. A physical therapist assistant positions a patient inside the parallel bars in preparation for gait training. When the parallel bars are positioned correctly, how many degrees of elbow flexion should the patient exhibit when standing erect?

    1. 5 – 15 degrees
    2. 15 – 25 degrees
    3. 30 – 40 degrees
    4. 40 – 50 degrees

16. A physical therapist assistant reviews a medical record to examine a patient's blood gas analysis. The medical record indicates that the patient's $PaCO_2$ is elevated and the pH is below normal levels. These findings are most representative of:

    1. respiratory acidosis
    2. respiratory alkalosis
    3. metabolic acidosis
    4. metabolic alkalosis

17. A physical therapist assistant monitors a 29-year-old male's vital signs during an exercise session. The patient has no known cardiovascular pathology and has been cleared for exercise by his physician. The patient's maximum heart rate during exercise should be calculated as:

    1. 170 beats per minute
    2. 180 beats per minute
    3. 191 beats per minute
    4. 201 beats per minute

18. A physical therapist assistant records the vital signs of a 42-year-old male before beginning an exercise program. The therapist determines that the patient's respiration rate and pulse rate are within normal limits. If the therapist expresses the value as a ratio of respiratory rate to pulse rate, which of the following would be considered normal?

    1. 1:5
    2. 1:3
    3. 4:1
    4. 6:1

19. A physical therapist assistant observes a patient's sputum sample. The therapist describes the color of the sample as yellow. Which condition is most likely associated with a yellow sputum sample?

   1. pulmonary edema
   2. neoplasm
   3. infection
   4. pneumonia

20. A physical therapist assistant completes a pulmonary function test on a patient diagnosed with chronic obstructive pulmonary disease. Which pulmonary measurement is defined as the amount of air that can be exhaled following a maximal inspiratory effort?

   1. total lung capacity
   2. functional residual capacity
   3. tidal volume
   4. vital capacity

II. *Intervention*

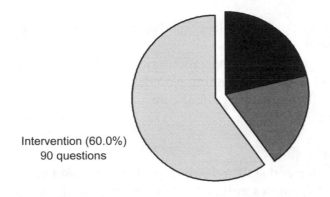

Intervention (60.0%)
90 questions

Intervention	Number of Questions
Non-procedural Intervention	28
Procedural Intervention	
Group I	16
Group II	17
Group III	20
Group IV	9
	Total = 90

Non-procedural Interventions

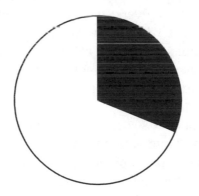

Non-procedural Intervention
28 questions

Non-procedural interventions

Coordination of Care
Included are the critical knowledge and skills related to coordination of care in accordance with the PT plan of care:
Communication with PT including organization/prioritization of information to be relayed to the PT and discharge planning with the PT
Progressing patient's treatment within plan of care
Directing tasks to support personnel

Interpersonal Communication
Included are critical knowledge and skills related to adjusting method of communication for patient/family/caregiver level of understanding and/or communication deficits:
Communicating with patients/families/caregivers and others
Communicating with PT and other health care providers
Communicating the role of the PT and PTA

Documentation
Included are critical knowledge and skills related to:
Reviewing medical charts
Objectively documenting results of tests and measures
Objectively documenting all aspects of care (including interventions, patient response to treatment, patient progress and outcomes)
Knowledge of medical and physical therapy terminology

Patient/Family/Client-related Instructions
Demonstrating and explaining treatment procedure, purpose, indication, contraindication, and precautions
Instructing and demonstrating safe application of patient care techniques performed with patient and family/caregivers, such as bed mobility, transfers, gait (with or without assistive devices), wheelchair setup, etc.
Providing written instructions to the patient/caregivers, as appropriate
Determining the effectiveness of the instruction and modifying, as needed
Selecting the appropriate teaching environment

Educational theories and patient's social and cultural background
Educational theories and interventions to achieve desired goal in patient education
Considering the patient's developmental level, cultural background, social history, home situation, and geographic barriers, etc.

Sample Questions

21. A physical therapist assistant demonstrates a lower extremity stretching exercise to a patient. To ensure the patient is able to complete the exercise, the therapist should:

    1. ask the patient to perform the exercise
    2. describe the exercise to the patient's spouse
    3. ask the patient to describe the exercise
    4. provide written instructions which describe the exercise

22. A physical therapist assistant completes lower extremity range of motion activities with a patient status post spinal cord injury. While performing the activity, the therapist notices that the patient's urine is extremely dark and has a distinctive foul smelling odor. The most appropriate action is to:

    1. verbally report the observation to the patient's physician
    2. verbally report the observation to the patient's nurse
    3. document and verbally report the observation to the patient's nurse
    4. document and verbally report the observation to the director of rehabilitation

23. A physical therapist assistant continually makes errors when completing daily documentation. Which of the following statements would be the most appropriate advice to the therapist when an error occurs?

    1. use correction fluid as needed on your documentation
    2. place a single line through the error, write "error", date, and initial it
    3. use pencil when completing your documentation
    4. use erasable ink when completing your documentation

24. A physical therapist assistant discusses risk factors associated with coronary artery disease with a patient in a phase I cardiac rehabilitation program. Which of the following risk factors is not modifiable?

    1. family history of coronary artery disease
    2. elevated serum cholesterol levels
    3. hypertension
    4. sedentary lifestyle

25. A physical therapist assistant presents an inservice entitled "Principles of Body Mechanics" to a group of certified nursing assistants. Which of the following principles would not be helpful for the group?

1. Avoid twisting your body when you lift.
2. Use longer lever arms for better control and efficiency when lifting or carrying.
3. When possible, push, pull, or roll an object rather than lift it.
4. Maintain your body's center of gravity close to the object's center of gravity when lifting.

26. A physical therapist assistant instructs a nine-year-old boy in a home exercise program. As the therapist starts to explain the exercise instructions, it becomes obvious that the boy is not interested. Which of the following would be the most beneficial action to improve compliance with the home exercise program?

1. Tell the boy he can leave because it is very difficult to help someone who does not want to be helped.
2. Continue with the instructions hoping that the boy is a better listener than he appears to be.
3. Lecture the boy on the importance of compliance with the home program.
4. Ask a family member to come into the room while you explain the home program.

27. A physical therapist assistant discusses total hip replacement precautions with a patient prior to surgery. Which of the following actions would best facilitate compliance with the precautions?

1. provide written materials outlining each precaution
2. discuss the precautions with the patient's spouse
3. ask the patient to repeat each precaution
4. tell the patient the precautions are very important

28. A patient eight days status post right total hip replacement loses his balance and falls to the ground. The patient is visibly shaken by the fall, but insists that he is uninjured. A physical therapist assistant assesses the right hip and although active motion elicits pain, all other findings are inconclusive. The most immediate action is to:

    1. continue with the current treatment so the patient does not focus on the incident
    2. notify the supervising physical therapist about the incident
    3. contact a physician to examine the patient
    4. gradually resume prior treatment

29. A patient rehabilitating from a motor vehicle accident complains that his pain medication is overdue. The most appropriate physical therapist assistant action is to:

    1. administer the patient's pain medication
    2. ask the patient to focus on the treatment session and not the pain
    3. notify the nursing staff of the patient's complaint
    4. document the patient's complaint in the medical record

30. A patient scheduled to undergo thoracic surgery is given preoperative instructions. During the training session the patient seems very discouraged and anxious about the impending surgery. The most appropriate mechanism to offer emotional support is to:

    1. tell the patient he will do just fine
    2. notify family members of the patient's present state
    3. visit the patient immediately after surgery
    4. listen to the patient express his feelings

Procedural Interventions

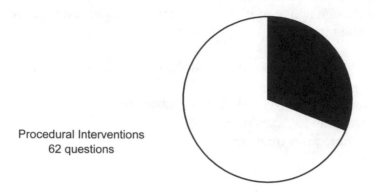

Procedural Interventions
62 questions

Procedural Interventions: Group I

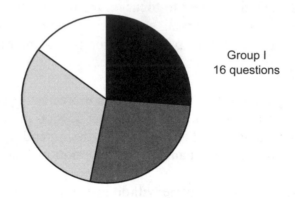

Group I
16 questions

Group I: Exercise and Manual Therapy

Exercise
    Aerobic capacity training/cardiovascular training
    Strengthening muscular endurance
    Stretching/range of motion
    Neuromuscular reeducation (including perceptual training)
    Balance/coordination
    Breathing
    Aquatic
    Postural
    Developmental

Manual Therapy
   Techniques of peripheral mobilization (extremities only at the beginning of joint
      range and not at high velocity)
   Techniques of soft tissue mobilization
   Techniques of manual traction

Sample Questions

31. A physical therapist assistant teaches a patient positioned in supine to
    posteriorly rotate his pelvis. The patient has full active and passive range
    of motion in the upper extremities, but is unable to achieve full shoulder
    flexion while maintaining the posterior pelvic tilt. Which of the following
    could best explain the patient's findings?

    1. capsular tightness
    2. latissimus dorsi tightness
    3. pectoralis minor tightness
    4. quadratus lumborum tightness

32. A patient eight weeks status post myocardial infarction is involved in a
    phase II cardiac rehabilitation program at a local hospital. What event
    usually signifies the completion of a phase II program?

    1. echocardiogram
    2. initiation of a high level aerobic exercise program
    3. low level treadmill test
    4. maximal treadmill test

33. A patient in a work hardening program is required to lift packages,
    weighing approximately 30 pounds, overhead to a conveyor belt. The
    patient can complete the task, but is unable to prevent excessive lumbar
    hyperextension while reaching for the conveyor belt. Which of the
    following conclusions is most accurate?

    1. additional weight should be added to the packages which will promote
       lumbar stability
    2. the patient should continue to lift the packages because they will
       gradually become stronger
    3. the task is too easy for the patient
    4. the task is too difficult for the patient

34. A physical therapist assistant implements a resistive program utilizing DeLorme and Watkins isotonic training program. The program is designed to strengthen the hamstrings and requires the patient to complete three sets of 10 repetitions. If the therapist determines the patient's ten repetition maximum is eighty pounds, how much weight would the patient be instructed to use on the first set?

1. 20 lbs.
2. 40 lbs.
3. 60 lbs.
4. 80 lbs.

35. A physical therapist assistant instructs a patient in frontal plane range of motion exercises. Which of the following exercises would be indicated?

1. shoulder flexion and extension
2. shoulder abduction and adduction
3. shoulder medial and lateral rotation
4. elbow flexion and extension

36. A physical therapist assistant uses therapeutic massage on a patient diagnosed with a hamstrings strain. The therapist can sense that the patient is unsure of what to expect during the massage. The most appropriate massage technique to initiate treatment is:

1. effleurage
2. petrissage
3. tapotement
4. vibration

37. A physical therapist assistant reviews safe exercise intensity parameters for a phase I inpatient cardiac rehabilitation program. Which parameter would be the most appropriate for the phase I program?

1. a maximum heart rate increase of 20 beats per minute above resting
2. a maximum heart rate increase of 30 beats per minute above resting
3. a maximum heart rate increase of 40 beats per minute above resting
4. a maximum heart rate increase of 50 beats per minute above resting

38. A physical therapist assistant treats a patient for a physical therapist on vacation. While completing a resistive exercise it becomes obvious that the patient cannot lift the selected weight. The most appropriate therapist action is to:

    1. discontinue the exercise session
    2. select a lighter weight
    3. ask the patient to attempt to lift the weight again
    4. attempt to contact the physical therapist and discuss the situation

39. A physical therapist assistant assists a patient rehabilitating from shoulder surgery with Codman's pendulum exercises. While performing the exercises the patient begins to experience back pain. The most appropriate modified patient position would be:

    1. supine
    2. standing
    3. sidelying
    4. prone

40. A patient diagnosed with peripheral vascular disease is treated in physical therapy. Which of the following objective findings would result in an ambulation exercise being contraindicated?

    1. decreased peripheral pulses
    2. resting claudication
    3. increased resting systolic blood pressure
    4. decreased lower extremity strength

Procedural Interventions: Group II

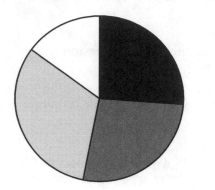

Group II
17 questions

Group II: Transfer and functional activities, gait training, assistive and adaptive devices, and modification of the environment

Transfer activities and functional activities, including safety related transfers
 Performing transfers
 Performing functional activities and training

Gait training and use of gait assistive devices (use of assistive devices with consideration of proper weight bearing status, gait deviations, balance deficits, components of gait cycle including pre-gait activities)

Application, adjustment and training in the use of devices and equipment, modification of the environment
 Adaptive devices
 Assistive devices
 Orthotic devices
 Prosthetic devices
 Protective devices
 Supportive devices, e.g., slings, compression garments, and supplemental oxygen
 Modification of environment for home/work/leisure activities

Sample Questions

41. A physical therapist assistant assesses a patient for a standard wheelchair. The therapist measures from the patient's posterior buttocks along the lateral thigh to the popliteal fold. The therapist then subtracts two inches from the measurement. This method can be used to measure:

    1. seat height
    2. seat depth
    3. seat width
    4. armrest length

42. A physical therapist assistant prepares a patient recovering from a total hip replacement for discharge from the hospital. The patient is 65-years-old and resides alone. Assuming an uncomplicated recovery, which piece of adaptive equipment would not be necessary for home use?

    1. long handled shoehorn
    2. raised toilet seat
    3. sliding board
    4. tub bench

43. When observing a patient ambulating, a physical therapist assistant notes that the patient's gait has the following characteristics: narrow base of support, short step length bilaterally, and decreased trunk rotation. This gait pattern is often observed in patients with a diagnosis of:

    1. stroke
    2. Parkinson's disease
    3. post-polio syndrome
    4. multiple sclerosis

44. A patient rehabilitating from injuries sustained in a motor vehicle accident is referred to physical therapy for gait training with an appropriate assistive device. The physical therapist assistant attempts to instruct the patient using axillary crutches, but feels the assistive device does not offer the patient enough stability or support. Which of the following assistive devices would be the most appropriate for the patient?

    1. walker
    2. cane
    3. Lofstrand crutches
    4. parallel bars

45. A physical therapist assistant transports a patient with left hemiplegia outside of the hospital in a wheelchair. In order to descend a curb using a backward approach, the therapist should position themselves:

    1. on the left side of the wheelchair
    2. on the right side of the wheelchair
    3. in front of the wheelchair
    4. in back of the wheelchair

46. A physical therapist assistant instructs a patient how to fall safely to the floor when using axillary crutches. Which of the following should be the first to occur in the case of a forward fall?

    1. reach toward the floor
    2. turn your face toward one side
    3. release the crutches
    4. flex the trunk and head

47. A physical therapist assistant instructs a patient rehabilitating from a tibial plateau fracture to ascend a curb using axillary crutches. The patient is partial weight bearing and uses a three-point gait pattern when ambulating. When ascending a curb the therapist should instruct the patient to lead with:

    1. the uninvolved lower extremity
    2. the involved lower extremity
    3. the crutches
    4. one crutch and the involved lower extremity

48. A physical therapist assistant instructs a patient how to rise from a chair before beginning ambulation activities with a walker. Which of the following instructions would be helpful to the patient?

    1. place both hands on the walker and pull yourself to a standing position
    2. push up on the chair with one hand and place the other hand on the edge of the walker for balance
    3. push up on the chair with both hands and reach for the walker once you are standing
    4. push up on the chair with both hands and reach for the walker while rising

49. A physical therapist assistant treats a patient that is unable to bear weight through the wrists and hands and has poor standing balance. The most appropriate assistive device for the patient is:

    1. axillary crutches with forearm attachments
    2. Lofstrand crutches
    3. a rolling walker
    4. a walker with platform attachments

50. A patient uses a wheelchair that has excessive seat depth. Which of the following is most likely to result when using the wheelchair?

    1. decreased trunk stability
    2. difficulty propelling the wheelchair
    3. difficulty transferring into the chair
    4. increased pressure in the popliteal area

Procedural Interventions: Group III

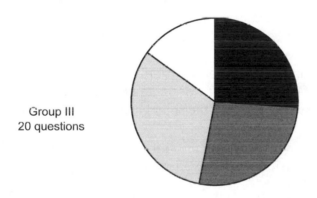

Group III
20 questions

Group III: Physical agents and modalities

Intermittent compression
Superficial thermotherapy, e.g., hot packs, paraffin, and cryotherapy
Ultrasound including phonophoresis
Electrical stimulation including iontophoresis
Biofeedback
Mechanical modalities: traction, tilt table/standing frames, continuous passive motion
Whirlpool/Hubbard tank

Sample Questions

51. A 45-year-old female with psoriasis is referred to physical therapy. The patient has several lesions on the posterior portion of her thigh extending into the popliteal fossa. The most appropriate therapeutic modality to treat the patient's condition is:

    1. iontophoresis
    2. moist heat
    3. ultrasound
    4. ultraviolet

52. A physical therapist assistant develops a home exercise program for a patient with acute Achilles tendonitis. As part of the program, the therapist would like to reduce the inflammation in the involved region. Which of the following modalities would be the most beneficial to achieve the therapist's goal?

    1. continuous ultrasound
    2. pulsed ultrasound
    3. ice massage
    4. whirlpool

53. A physical therapist assistant administers ultrasound over a patient's anterior thigh. After one minute of treatment the patient reports feeling a slight burning sensation under the sound head. The therapist's most appropriate action is to:

    1. explain to the patient that what he feels is not out of the ordinary when using ultrasound
    2. decrease the intensity of the ultrasound and continue to monitor the patient's response
    3. discontinue treatment and contact the referring physician
    4. continue with treatment utilizing the current parameters

54. A 78-year-old male, one month status post open reduction and internal fixation of an intertrochanteric fracture is referred to physical therapy. The patient has pain with active movement and decreased hip range of motion. Which of the following modalities would be contraindicated for the patient?

    1. moist heat
    2. continuous ultrasound
    3. cryotherapy
    4. shortwave diathermy

55. A physical therapy department develops guidelines for electrical equipment care and service. Which of the following guidelines does not meet acceptable equipment care and service standards?

    1. AC power receptacles and plugs should be hospital grade quality
    2. electrical equipment should be inspected every 24-36 months
    3. a file of clinical and technical information for each piece of equipment should be established
    4. documentation of inspection and repair activities should be available for each device

56. A physical therapist assistant uses iontophoresis to treat a patient diagnosed with lateral epicondylitis. Which type of current would be the most appropriate?

    1. direct
    2. alternating
    3. pulsatile
    4. interferential

57. A physical therapist assistant utilizes a TENS unit to treat a patient rehabilitating from a laminectomy. Immediately after turning on the current, the patient begins to experience severe discomfort in the lumbar spine. The most appropriate therapist action is to:

    1. decrease the pulse width
    2. increase the pulse frequency
    3. increase the ramp time
    4. turn off the current

58. A physical therapist assistant treats an obese patient referred to physical therapy with a hip flexor strain. Which modality would have the greatest ability to elevate the temperature of fatty tissue to potentially dangerous levels?

    1. diathermy
    2. hot packs
    3. paraffin
    4. ultraviolet

59. A physical therapist assistant applies a hot pack to the low back of a patient diagnosed with myofascial pain syndrome. Which patient position would most accelerate the rate of heat transfer?

    1. left sidelying
    2. right sidelying
    3. prone
    4. supine

60. Results of an x-ray of the shoulder reveal areas of calcium deposits in a patient with diffuse shoulder pain. Based on the diagnostic finding, the physician refers the patient to physical therapy for iontophoresis treatment. Which medication would be the most useful to incorporate during iontophoresis treatment?

    1. acetic acid
    2. salicylates
    3. lidocaine
    4. zinc oxide

Procedural Interventions: Group IV

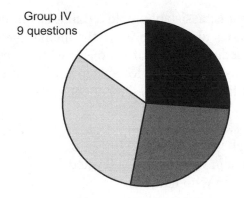

Group IV
9 questions

Group IV: Airway clearance techniques, wound care, promoting health and wellness (includes some components of non-procedural intervention), and intervention effectiveness

Airway clearance techniques
    Breathing strategies, e.g., coughing, huffing, and pacing
    Manual/mechanical techniques, e.g., percussion, vibration, suctioning
    Positioning

Wound care and skin integrity
    Skin status monitoring
    Patient positioning and use of adaptive/protective equipment for pressure relief
    Dressing application and removal
    Topical agent application
    Debridement techniques excluding sharp debridement

Intervention effectiveness - modify intervention based on patient response

Promoting health and wellness and prevention, including instructions and intervention

61. A physical therapist assistant employed in a hospital treats a 67-year-old male with a venous ulcer posterior to the medial malleolus. The patient has a lengthy medical history of venous insufficiency including admission to the hospital six months ago for a deep venous thrombosis. Which finding is most likely based on the patient's condition?

    1 pale, white skin color
    2. absent peripheral pulses
    3. diminished pain with the legs elevated
    4. thin, shiny skin with hair loss

62. A physical therapist assistant discusses general guidelines for prevention of pressure ulcers with a patient during a whirlpool treatment. Which statement is the most accurate?

    1. massage over bony prominences to promote circulation
    2. reposition while in bed every 3-4 hours
    3. use a "doughnut-type" ring when sitting for long periods of time
    4. eat a balanced diet that is high in protein, vitamins, and minerals

The following figure should be used to answer question 63:

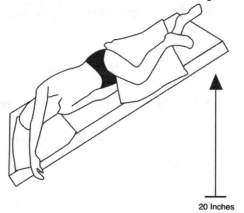

20 Inches

63. A 16-year-old patient requires chest physical therapy due to cystic fibrosis. Prior to implementing the intervention the physical therapist assistant positions the patient as shown above. This position would be most appropriate for the:

    1. lingula segment of the left upper lobe
    2. right middle lobe
    3. anterior basal segment of the left lower lobe
    4. superior segment of the right lower lobe

64. A physical therapist assistant applies a custom fabricated hand splint to a patient that sustained a burn to his right wrist and hand. The splint maintains the wrist in extension; the metacarpophalangeal joints in 75 degrees of flexion; the proximal and distal interphalangeal joints in flexion; and the thumb in abduction. Based on the supplied description of the splint, which area would be most susceptible to contracture?

   1. wrist
   2. metacarpophalangeal joints
   3. proximal and distal interphalangeal joints
   4. thumb

65. A 32-year-old female is admitted to the hospital after sustaining extensive burns to her trunk and right upper extremity. Which of the following burn classifications would most likely require the use of a graft?

   1. superficial burn
   2. superficial partial-thickness burn
   3. deep partial-thickness burn
   4. full-thickness burn

66. A physical therapist assistant begins gait training with a patient who recently received an ankle-foot orthosis to assist with foot drop and sensory loss. A reddened area over the lateral malleolus persists after ambulating sixty feet. The most appropriate therapist response is to:

   1. direct the patient to wear the orthosis at all times because the body will eventually get used to it
   2. direct the patient to make an appointment with the orthotist and continue to wear the orthosis until that time
   3. direct the patient not to wear the orthosis until modifications are made
   4. direct the patient to make an appointment with the physician

67. An order for chest physical therapy is received for an 82-year-old female. The patient recently underwent surgery for a hip fracture and has been taking Coumadin postoperatively. She has a history of multiple compression fractures of thoracic vertebrae. The greatest caution should be taken in the administration of:

   1. diaphragmatic breathing exercises
   2. postural drainage
   3. therapeutic percussion
   4. pursed-lip breathing

68. A physical therapist assistant prepares to apply a sterile dressing to a wound after debridement. The therapist begins the process by drying the wound using a towel. The therapist applies medication to the wound using a gauze pad and then applies a series of dressings, which are secured using a bandage. Application of which of the following would not require the use of sterile technique?

1. bandage
2. dressings
3. medication
4. towel

69. A physical therapist assistant instructs a patient's spouse to remove and reapply a bandage. Which of the following instructional methods would be the most appropriate to ensure the task is performed appropriately?

1. have the patient instruct the spouse how to remove and reapply the bandage
2. provide written instructions on how to remove and reapply the bandage
3. instruct the spouse to remove and reapply the bandage and observe her performance
4. instruct the spouse to contact the physical therapy department if she has specific questions

70. A physical therapist assistant applies a bandage to secure a dressing over a wound on the forearm. Which of the following would indicate that the bandage was applied too loosely?

1. the distal segment appears to be pale
2. edema develops in the distal segment
3. the bandage changes position with active movement
4. the patient complains of pain in the segment distal to the bandage

III. *Standards of Care*

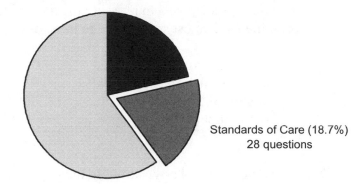

Standards of Care (18.7%)
28 questions

Standards of Care

Patient Confidentiality, Autonomy and Consent
    Maintaining patient confidentiality
    Maintaining patient autonomy and obtaining consent

Work Parameters
    Work under the direction and supervision of a PT in an ethical, legal, and effective
        manner
    Knowing and working within state law and rules governing physical therapy
    Performing only those tasks that are within the PTAs knowledge and skill level
    Utilizing clinical decision making in data collection and interventions

Body Mechanics/positioning
    Body mechanics (utilize, teach, reinforce, observe)
    Positioning, draping, and stabilization

Safety, CPR, Emergency Care, First Aid
    Ensuring patient safety and safe application of patient care
    Performing first aid
    Performing emergency procedures
    Performing CPR

Standard Precautions
    Sterile procedures
    Demonstrating appropriate sequencing of events related to universal precautions
    Demonstrating aseptic techniques
    Properly discarding soiled items
    Determining equipment to be used and assembling all materials, sterile and non-
        sterile

71. A patient predisposed to pressure ulcers is placed in supine. Which bony prominence is most susceptible to breakdown in this position?

    1. tip of the acromion
    2. posterior iliac crest
    3. dorsum of the foot
    4. ischial tuberosity

72. A twelve-year-old boy, sitting in the physical therapy waiting area, suddenly grasps his throat and appears to be in distress. The boy slowly stands, but is obviously unable to breathe. The therapist recognizing the signs of an airway obstruction should administer:

    1. abdominal thrusts
    2. chest thrusts
    3. back blows
    4. back blows in combination with abdominal thrusts

73. A patient with a lengthy cardiac history ambulates on a treadmill as part of a phase II cardiac rehabilitation program. Suddenly, the patient begins to experience signs of an angina attack. The physical therapist assistant's most immediate response should be to:

    1. contact emergency medical services
    2. stop the exercise session
    3. contact the patient's physician
    4. document the incident in the medical record

74. A patient sustains a deep laceration on the right thigh after falling into a modality cart. The laceration causes immediate and excessive bleeding. The physical therapist assistant should first:

    1. apply direct pressure over the laceration
    2. assess the lower extremity
    3. put on gloves
    4. contact the supervising physical therapist

75. A patient that has been on extended bed rest is positioned on a tilt table. After slightly elevating the head of the tilt table, the patient begins to demonstrate signs of orthostatic hypotension. The physical therapist assistant's most immediate response should be to:

    1. reassure the patient that the response is not unusual
    2. contact the supervising physical therapist for assistance
    3. document the incident in the patient's chart
    4. lower the tilt table

76. A patient rehabilitating from a fractured humerus has completed six weeks of physical therapy and is ready to be discharged with a home exercise program. The patient is extremely pleased with his progress in therapy and gives the therapist a check for $50.00 as a token of his appreciation. The most appropriate therapist action is to:

    1. accept the money
    2. donate the money to charity
    3. donate the money to the department's general expense fund
    4. explain to the patient that you are not permitted to accept money

77. A physical therapist assistant can be liable for the use of a patient's medical record without receiving prior patient consent. Which of the following situations may not require patient consent?

    1. taking pictures of a patient during treatment
    2. videotaping a patient's gait
    3. research where anonymity is preserved
    4. permitting an unauthorized person access to a patient's medical record

78. A physical therapist requests that a physical therapist assistant treat a patient diagnosed with a temporomandibular joint disorder. The physical therapist assistant has limited clinical experience with the diagnosis and is therefore quite apprehensive. The most appropriate physical therapist assistant response is to:

    1. attempt to treat the patient
    2. discuss the situation with the supervising physical therapist
    3. ask another physical therapist assistant to treat the patient
    4. refuse to treat the patient

79. A physical therapist assistant waiting for her next patient to arrive, observes another patient ambulating independently in the parallel bars. The patient appears to lack the necessary strength and coordination required to complete the activity. The therapist's most immediate response would be to:

1. inform the patient's therapist of her observation
2. assist the patient back to a chair and contact the patient's therapist
3. ask the patient if they need assistance
4. continue to observe the patient, but do not interfere

80. A physical therapist assistant provides patient coverage for a physical therapist on vacation. The physical therapist assistant should be allowed to perform all of the following except:

1. supervise exercise activities
2. modify the plan of care
3. gait training activities
4. write daily progress notes

Conclusion

Candidates should attempt to generate their own interpretation of each category and subcategory of the content outline and speculate on what type of questions could be asked. By doing this, candidates will acquire a deeper and more comprehensive understanding of the material on the Physical Therapist Assistant Examination.

Answer Key

1. Answer: 3   Resource: Anderson (p. 957)
   Kinesthesia is defined as the ability to perceive extent, direction, or weight of movement.

2. Answer: 3   Resource: Norkin (p. 26)
   Since the 15 is to the left of 0 it is indicative of hyperextension, therefore 150 + 15 = 165.

3. Answer: 4   Resource: Minor (p. 134)
   Active-assistive exercise requires movement performed by a patient with additional movement or mechanical assistance.

4. Answer: 3   Resource: Hoppenfeld (p. 106)
   The hyoid bone is located at the same level as the C3 vertebral body. The thyroid cartilage is directly below the hyoid bone.

5. Answer: 1   Resource: Norkin (p. 9)
   Structures capable of producing firm end-feels when stretched include muscle, capsule and ligaments.

6. Answer: 1   Resource: Hoppenfeld (p. 216)
   The sinus tarsi area is located immediately anterior to the lateral malleolus. The soft tissue depression consists of a tunnel between the calcaneus and talus. The anterior talofibular ligament is often the first ligament affected by an inversion ankle injury.

7. Answer: 1   Resource: Norkin (p. 142)
   The typical end-feel associated with knee flexion is soft due to contact between the muscles of the posterior calf and thigh or between the heel and buttocks.

8. Answer: 1   Resource: Norkin (p. 162)
   Motion occurring at the subtalar joint should be measured with the moving arm of the goniometer positioned over the posterior midline of the calcaneus. Ankle complex inversion and eversion can be measured with the moving arm positioned over the anterior midline of the second metatarsal.

9. Answer: 2   Resource: Hertling (p. 85)
   Sensory testing for light touch is performed by applying the piece of cotton to selected dermatomes and asking the patient when the sensation is perceived.

10. Answer: 1   Resource: Kendall (p. 187)
A muscle grade of poor requires a given muscle to be tested in a gravity
eliminated position. A supine position would best limit the effects of gravity on
the hip adductors.

11. Answer: 2   Resource: O'Sullivan (p. 848)
A superficial partial-thickness burn involves both the epidermis and a portion of
the dermis. Healing typically occurs in approximately three weeks with little or
no scarring.

12. Answer: 4   Resource: Waxman (p. 230)
The vestibular system is responsible for the maintenance of stance and body
posture, coordination of body, head and eye movements, and visual fixation.
Symptoms of possible vestibular dysfunction include nystagmus, vertigo, and
ataxia.

13. Answer: 4   Resource: Brannon (p. 316)
Facial color, expression, and rating on a perceived exertion scale are considered
subjective measures of endurance.

14. Answer: 4   Resource: Pierson (p. 57)
The width of a bladder should be approximately 40% of the circumference of the
midpoint of the limb. Bladder width for an average size adult is 5-6 inches.

15. Answer: 2   Resource: Pierson (p. 195)
A patient should exhibit 15 - 25 degrees of elbow flexion while standing upright
and grasping the parallel bars six inches anterior to the hips.

16. Answer: 1   Resource: Irwin (p. 348)
Respiratory acidosis is caused by retention of carbon dioxide due to pulmonary
insufficiency. Signs and symptoms include dizziness, tingling, and syncope.

17. Answer: 3   Resource: Minor (p. 39)
Age predicted maximum heart rate = 220 - age. Maximum heart rate = 220 - 29 = 191.

18. Answer: 1   Resource: Minor (p. 39)
Although normal values deviate from source to source, broad ranges of normal
values for respiration rate and heart rate are as follows: respiration rate 12-18
breaths/minute, heart rate 60-100 beats per minute.

19. Answer: 3   Resource: Rothstein (p. 533)
Yellow or greenish sputum is commonly associated with acute or chronic
infection.

20. Answer: 4   Resource: Goodman – Pathology (p. 854)
Vital Capacity = Inspiratory Reserve Volume + Tidal Volume + Expiratory
Reserve Volume. Vital capacity can be measured using a spirometer.

21. Answer: 1   Resource: Haggard (p. 112)
Having a patient perform a selected exercise not only provides information on if he/she
can successfully complete the exercise, but also presents the therapist with an opportunity
to provide feedback.

22. Answer: 3   Resource: Pierson (p. 267)
Any change in color or odor of urine is significant and should therefore be reported and
documented.

23. Answer: 2   Resource: Kettenbach (p. 10)
When an error occurs in the medical record the most appropriate method is to
place a single line through the error, write "error", and date and initial it.
Therapists should avoid using "white out " or trying to conceal a mistake.

24. Answer: 1   Resource: Irwin (p. 8)
A positive family history of coronary artery disease is a risk factor, however it is
not a modifiable risk factor.

25. Answer: 2   Resource: Kisner (p. 673)
Using a longer lever arm when lifting or carrying will place more pressure on the
spine and hips and is biomechanically less efficient.

26. Answer: 4   Resource: Purtilo (p. 292)
Due to the patient's age it would be appropriate to ask a family member to come into the
room. To reprimand the boy in any form may only serve to diminish compliance.

27. Answer: 1   Resource: Haggard (p. 84)
Preoperative instructions are often forgotten by patients by the time the surgical
procedure is performed. It is therefore important to provide the patient with some
form of written material so that the information can be revisited following
surgery.

28. Answer: 2   Resource: Guide for Conduct of the
                                            Physical Therapist Assistant
Since the therapist's findings were inconclusive and the patient is status post total
hip replacement it is necessary for the assistant to notify the supervising physical
therapist.

29. Answer: 3   Resource: Guide for Conduct of the
                                            Physical Therapist Assistant
The nursing staff is the appropriate party to assess the veracity of the patient's
complaint and if necessary administer the pain medication.

30. Answer: 4   Resource: Davis (p. 101)
Listening to the patient express his feelings demonstrates respect for his present emotional state. Actions to dismiss the patient's feelings are insensitive and can damage the patient-therapist relationship.

31. Answer: 2   Resource: Hoppenfeld (p. 279)
Shortening of the latissimus dorsi often presents as a limitation of shoulder flexion or abduction due to the muscles origin on the external lip of the iliac crest and its insertion on the intertubercular groove of the humerus.

32. Answer: 4   Resource: Irwin (p. 5)
A phase II cardiac rehabilitation program typically begins with a low level treadmill test and ends with a maximal treadmill test and cardiac catheterization.

33. Answer: 4   Resource: Kisner (p. 674)
The packages may be too heavy or the conveyor belt may be too high. In both cases the task is too difficult.

34. Answer: 2   Resource: Kisner (p. 125)
The first set consists of ten repetitions at 50% of the 10 repetition maximum. 10 RM = 80 pounds; 50% of 80 pounds = 40 pounds.

35. Answer: 2   Resource: Norkin (p. 5)
Motions in the frontal plane occur around an anterior-posterior axis. Abduction and adduction occur in the frontal plane.

36. Answer: 1   Resource: De Domenico (p. 9)
Effleurage is defined as passing the hands over a large body area through gentle or deep stroking. Effleurage is often used as an initial, transitional, and/or final massage technique.

37. Answer: 1   Resource: Brannon (p. 3)
A maximum heart rate increase of 20 beats per minute above resting is considered a safe guideline for a patient participating in a phase I program.

38. Answer: 2   Resource: Kisner (p. 98)
The patient may benefit from completing the exercise with the lighter weight. The patient's response to the exercise with the original weight and the lighter weight should be documented.

39. Answer: 4   Resource: Kisner (p. 364)
Codman's pendulum exercises can be performed with the patient in prone on a plinth with the arm over the side. It is not as desirable as a standing position since it is difficult to initiate movement using the trunk in the prone position.

40. Answer: 2   Resource: Kisner (p. 715)
    Patients with peripheral vascular disease that present with resting claudication are not
    considered candidates for ambulation exercise programs.

41. Answer: 2   Resource: Pierson (p. 149)
    The formula for seat depth subtracts two inches from the obtained measurement to
    avoid impingement on the vascular structures in the posterior aspect of the knee.
    Average seat depth is approximately 16 inches in an adult wheelchair.

42. Answer: 3   Resource: O'Sullivan (p. 336)
    A patient rehabilitating from a total hip replacement would not typically need to
    utilize a sliding board following surgery. The remaining adaptive devices are
    often necessary in the home due to the established hip precautions.

43. Answer: 2   Resource: Pauls (p. 343)
    The described gait pattern is characteristic of a patient with Parkinson's disease.
    Other symptoms associated with Parkinson's include postural instability, resting
    tremor, rigidity, and bradykinesia.

44. Answer: 1   Resource: Pierson (p. 193)
    A walker provides more stability than axillary crutches and is more functional
    than the parallel bars.

45. Answer: 4   Resource: Pierson (p. 170)
    The therapist should be positioned in back of the wheelchair in order to optimally
    protect the patient.

46. Answer: 3   Resource: Pierson (p. 248)
    The most immediate action should be to release the crutches. Failure to release
    the crutches will result in an inability to break the fall using the upper extremities.

47. Answer: 1   Resource: Minor (p. 309)
    When ascending a curb a patient should lead with the uninvolved lower extremity in
    order to avoid placing unnecessary force on the involved extremity.

48. Answer: 3   Resource: Minor (p. 314)
    Pushing up on the chair with both hands provides the most stable base to achieve
    a standing position. It is important not to reach for the walker while rising from
    the chair since the action may have a tendency to move the patient's center of
    gravity outside their base of support.

49. Answer: 4   Resource: Pierson (p. 193)
    The patient requires the stability offered by the walker, however also needs the
    platform attachments to avoid bearing weight through the wrists and hands.

50. Answer: 4   Resource: Pierson (p. 152)
    Excessive seat depth can lead to the front of the seat exerting pressure into the
    popliteal area. The pressure can lead to circulatory compromise and/or skin
    breakdown.

51. Answer: 4   Resource: Michlovitz (p. 272)
    Ultraviolet light is primarily used to treat dermatologic conditions including
    psoriasis.

52. Answer: 3   Resource: Michlovitz (p. 99)
    Ice massage is an accessible and effective cryotherapeutic agent that is often
    incorporated into a home exercise program to reduce inflammation.

53. Answer: 2   Resource: Michlovitz (p. 198)
    A patient report of a slight burning sensation under the soundhead can be due to
    inadequate coupling, loosening of the crystal, or hot spots due to a high beam
    nonuniformity ratio.

54. Answer: 4   Resource: Michlovitz (p. 233)
    Internal or external metal objects are contraindications for shortwave and microwave
    diathermy.

55. Answer: 2   Resource: Robinson (p. 75)
    Electrical equipment should be inspected at a minimum on an annual basis.

56. Answer: 1   Resource: Robinson (p. 335)
    Iontophoresis refers to the administration of ions through a membrane using direct
    current. Examples of medications used in iontophoresis include acetic acid,
    lidocaine, and dexamethasone.

57. Answer: 4   Resource: Robinson (p. 76)
    Severe discomfort should not be associated with the use of any electrical
    stimulation equipment.

58. Answer: 1   Resource: Michlovitz (p. 215)
    Diathermy is considered a deep heating agent while the remaining options are
    superficial heating agents.

59. Answer: 4   Resource: Michlovitz (p. 116)
    When lying on a hot pack in the supine position the rate of heat transfer to the low
    back is accelerated due to the influence of body weight.

60. Answer: 1   Resource: Cameron (p. 403)
    Iontophoresis refers to the delivery of ions into the tissue through the skin using
    electrical current. The acetate ion (negative polarity) in acetic acid has been
    shown to assist with reducing the size of calcium deposits.

61. Answer: 3   Resource: Goodman – Pathology
                                                (p. 463)
Elevation of the legs assists with venous return and therefore would tend to be
more comfortable for a patient with venous insufficiency. The remaining options
are more representative of signs and symptoms of an arterial ulcer.

62. Answer: 4   Resource: Anderson (p. 1318)
Repositioning in bed should occur at least every two hours. Massage should be
avoided over any bony prominence, however may occur in the surrounding area.
Doughnut rings are contraindicated for people at risk for breakdown because the
ring itself places extra pressure on the areas of contact.

63. Answer: 3   Resource: Brannon (p. 426)
Postural drainage to the anterior basal segments of the left lower lobe requires the
patient to be positioned on his right side and the foot of the bed elevated 18-20
inches.

64. Answer: 3   Resource: Goodman – Pathology
                                                (p. 307)
The proximal and distal interphalangeal joints are susceptible to a flexion
contracture when splinted in a flexed position. Correct positioning of PIPs and
DIPs would be in extension.

65. Answer: 4   Resource: Rothstein (p. 1117)
Full-thickness burns are characterized by complete destruction of the epidermis
and dermis with or without damage to the subcutaneous fat layer. Since new
tissue is only generated from the periphery of the burn site, grafts are necessary.

66. Answer: 3   Resource: Clark (p. 343)
Since the patient has a sensory alteration and ambulating a distance of only sixty
feet created irritation, it is advisable to avoid utilizing the orthosis until
modifications are made.

67. Answer: 3   Resource: Irwin (p. 345)
Percussion is a technique that can be used to mobilize retained secretions. The technique
involves direct contact over a given segment of the lung and should therefore be used
with caution based on the patient's past medical history.

68. Answer: 1   Resource: Pierson (p. 311)
A bandage is used to secure underlying dressing and therefore does not come in direct
contact with the wound.

69. Answer: 3   Resource: Haggard (p. 112)
Direct observation is the only method to ensure the task is performed appropriately.

70. Answer: 3   Resource: Pierson (p. 311)
    A change in position of a bandage with active movement indicates it is too loose
    and may need to be reapplied.

71. Answer: 2   Resource: Pierson (p. 33)
    Bony prominences susceptible to breakdown in the supine position include the
    spine, inferior angle of the scapula, the spinous processes of the vertebrae,
    posterior iliac crests, sacrum, and posterior calcaneus.

72. Answer: 1   Resource: Rothstein (p. 1218)
    Abdominal thrusts are indicated in the presence of a complete airway obstruction
    for individuals over one year of age.

73. Answer: 2   Resource: Brannon (p. 260)
    The therapist's most immediate response should be to stop the exercise session.
    Failure to stop the exercise session could result in an unsafe situation.

74. Answer: 3   Resource: Pierson (p. 281)
    The first and most appropriate action is to put on gloves. Although direct pressure over
    the laceration is necessary, a therapist must always protect him/herself first.

75. Answer: 4   Resource: Goodman-Pathology (p. 296)
    The most immediate response should be to eliminate the causative factor which is the
    positional change. Therefore, it is necessary to lower the tilt table.

76. Answer: 4   Resource: Guide for Conduct of the
                                             Physical Therapist Assistant
    The Code of Ethics states that "therapists seek reimbursement for their services that is
    deserved and reasonable." Accepting a check from a patient, regardless of its use is
    unacceptable.

77. Answer: 3   Resource: Currier (p. 67)
    There are some situations in which research can take place without patient
    consent. An example of this may involve a therapist compiling selected discharge
    data for patient's receiving total knee arthroplasty within the last two years.

78. Answer: 2   Resource: Standards of Ethical
                                             Conduct for the Physical
                                             Therapist Assistant
    The Standards of Ethical Conduct state that "Physical therapist assistants make those
    judgments that are commensurate with their qualifications as physical therapist
    assistants." This includes not only academic training, but also individual clinical
    experience.

79. Answer: 2

Resource: Guide for Conduct of the Physical Therapist Assistant

The therapist has made a judgment that the patient "lacks the necessary strength and coordination required to complete the activity independently." The only method to resolve the situation and be sure the patient is unharmed is to become directly involved.

80. Answer: 2

Resource: Guide to Physical Therapist Practice (p. S42)

Although physical therapist assistants may alter specific intervention procedures within an established plan of care as a result of a change in patient status, they are not able to modify the established plan.

Final Preparation

As the date of the Physical Therapist Assistant Examination steadily approaches, candidates usually experience an increase in their anxiety level. Candidates often voice concerns such as: "How am I going to remember everything?", "What if I studied the wrong material?" "Did I study enough?" Unfortunately, the answer to these seemingly simple questions can be very complicated.

The good news is that candidates who have taken the time to develop a comprehensive study plan and periodically assess their progress towards meeting established goals tend to perform well on the examination. The performance of candidates who have either neglected to study or have approached their studying in a random or inefficient manner can be much more difficult to predict.

Regardless of which description best describes your preparation, when the examination is less than 48 hours away, it is simply too late to make any significant changes in your study plan. Instead, candidates need to focus on other variables they can control. This unit will offer specific suggestions for candidates to incorporate into their final preparation.

Examination Strategy

Just as you developed an individualized study plan according to your needs as a learner, you now need to consider how you can take the examination with the same considerations in mind.

If you determined you were an Active/Active or Active/Passive learner for input and processing, you may find this three and one half hour, physically passive testing environment to be particularly trying and consequently, anxiety producing. You may find yourself being distracted by every noise, vibration, and movement in the room, and may notice that your ability to concentrate has been compromised. Although it is impossible to have the same type of control over the examination site as you did over your study sessions, it is possible to make a few alterations that can be beneficial:

1. Attempt to secure a corner location. Corner locations tend to limit peripheral vision distracters.
2. Consider wearing earplugs to block out some of the unnecessary background noise.
3. Prior to beginning the examination write down question numbers 25, 50, 75, 100, 125, and 150 on a piece of paper and place it in a visible location. As you progress through the examination, perform a brief relaxation exercise at each of the scheduled intervals. A sample relaxation exercise is outlined in the Appendix.

If you determined you were a Passive/Active or Passive/Passive learner you may not be as challenged by the physically passive nature of the three and one half hour testing environment, but the intensity of the mental activity may produce anxiety in the form of tense muscles and a gradual lengthening of the time needed to answer each question. Here are some recommendations you may consider:

1. Attempt to secure a location where you will not be disturbed by the movements of other candidates.
2. If you concentrate better in a quiet setting, you may want to consider wearing earplugs.
3. Prior to beginning the examination write down question number 50 and 100 on a piece of paper and place it in a visible location. As you progress through the examination, perform the relaxation exercise at each of the scheduled intervals. A sample relaxation exercise is outlined in the Appendix.

The suggested recommendations for each learning style should be incorporated into a candidate's study plan. Candidates can attempt to incorporate the recommendations as they take the 150 question sample examination located in Unit Eight. By utilizing this information prior to the actual examination, candidates can evaluate the utility of each suggestion and construct an individualized examination strategy.

Miscellaneous Items

Scheduling the Examination

Candidates will have 60 days from the date on the Federation of State Boards of Physical Therapy "approval to test" letter to take the Physical Therapist Assistant Examination. It is important to schedule an appointment relatively early in the 60 day window in order to ensure availability at a local Prometric Testing Center. Candidates should schedule their examination at a time consistent with their optimal level of functioning. For example, if a candidate tends to be a morning person it would be prudent to schedule the examination early in the morning. Candidates with significant anxiety related to the examination may also want an early appointment in order to avoid worrying about the examination throughout the day.

Examination Site

If candidates are not familiar with the exact location of the examination site, it is often prudent to travel to the site before the actual examination date. This trip can serve two important purposes. The first is that candidates will have an accurate idea of the time necessary to travel to the site, and therefore will be able to plan accordingly the day of the examination. The second purpose is that the pre-examination visit should eliminate the possibility of getting lost and subsequently being late for the examination.

Studying

Last minute studying is strongly discouraged. Candidates should avoid studying the entire day before the examination. A 24-hour period without studying is often necessary to put the mind at ease and limit needless worry about the examination. Candidates who have prepared adequately will feel comfortable with their preparation and will go into the examination with a high level of confidence. Last minute studying will only serve to undermine this confidence.

Testing Supplies

Take time the day prior to the examination to gather the necessary supplies. Read the information from the Prometric Testing Center carefully and be sure that you have secured and packed each of the items. Failure to provide a given item, such as two forms of identification, can result in a scheduled appointment being delayed or canceled.

Dress

Plan to dress comfortably for the examination. Select an outfit the night before that can be altered depending on conditions at the examination site. Generally a blouse or shirt with a sweater can accommodate for a variety of conditions. Pants are generally the preferred choice over shorts. Light pants tend to be comfortable in warm weather and also keep the chill off in air conditioning or colder conditions. Although your clothing will not determine your examination score, it is important to be comfortable. Excessive heat or cold can serve as a distracter during the examination.

Entertainment

The night before the examination, engage in an activity that you particularly enjoy, whether it's going to your favorite restaurant, a theater performance, or spending a quiet evening at home with your significant other. By taking part in a planned activity, you will avoid focusing on the impending examination and harness any growing anxiety.

Bedtime

Make a special effort to be in bed at or before your usual time. Your mind will need to be rested and at an optimal functioning level the day of the examination. Lack of sleep or other deterrents, such as alcohol or drugs will serve to limit your performance. Use an alarm clock to make sure you are up in plenty of time on the big day.

The Big Day

As the blare of the alarm clock breaks the morning calm, your day officially begins. Since you already have performed the majority of the tasks associated with the examination, there should be little extra to do except your routine daily activities.

Special attention should be given to eating well balanced meals. Considering there will be some travel associated with getting to the examination site, and the allotted examination time is three and one half hours, it may be quite awhile until you have the opportunity to eat again.

Travel

Be sure to leave extra time when traveling to the Prometric Testing Center. Leaving additional time will allow a candidate to enter the examination site calm and collected. Arriving late or just as the examination is scheduled to begin will cause needless stress and may have a negative impact on a candidate's performance.

Show Time

Always take the available time to review the tutorial prior to beginning the examination. The fifteen minutes allotted to the tutorial does not count toward the three and one half hour time period given to take the actual examination. Be sure that you have a thorough understanding of the information conveyed in the tutorial prior to beginning the examination. If anything remains unclear, seek additional guidance from an authorized agent at the testing center. The tutorial not only reminds you of several important features of computer based testing, but can also serve as a way to limit growing test anxiety.

When taking the actual examination, read all questions carefully and consider each option with an open mind. Finish the examination only when you either have used all of the allotted time or have finished answering all of the questions. When leaving the examination take solace knowing that you did the best job possible. Take pride in the fact your preparation was both timely and effective. Resist the temptation to scrutinize and second guess yourself; it will only result in wasted energy and cannot possibly change your examination results. Typically, candidates will be notified of their results in 3-10 days by their state licensing agency.

Conclusion

We have presented a number of different strategies that, when used appropriately, can assist candidates to maximize their performance on the Physical Therapist Assistant Examination. Candidates should avoid focusing on any of the specific strategies in isolation, and instead incorporate them into a comprehensive study plan. By utilizing the information contained in the text and developing specific individual strategies, you already have taken a large step towards being successful on the Physical Therapist Assistant Examination.

Sample Examination

As we have indicated numerous times throughout this text, candidates can obtain a great deal of valuable information by taking sample examinations. Candidates who are exposed to sample examinations have several distinct opportunities that otherwise may not be available.

1. Candidates have the opportunity to refine their test taking skills with sample questions that are similar in design and format to actual examination questions.

2. Candidates have the opportunity to assess their current level of preparation prior to the actual examination.

In this unit, candidates will have the opportunity to take a 150 question sample examination. In order to assess a candidate's performance on the sample examination, a number of indicators must be examined. Perhaps the most obvious indicator is the number of questions a candidate answers correctly. Since the Physical Therapist Assistant Examination consists of 150 scored items, the maximum number of questions a candidate can answer correctly is 150. The established criterion-referenced score for the 150 question sample examination is 112.

Unfortunately, it is not possible to identify a single number of questions that must be answered correctly in order to be successful on the actual Physical Therapist Assistant Examination. This number fluctuates based on the level of difficulty of each given examination. Candidates should use the number of questions answered correctly on the sample examination only as a general indicator of their current level of preparation.

There are a number of less obvious indicators that can offer candidates feedback as they prepare for the Physical Therapist Assistant Examination. These indicators often are best examined by answering several selected questions.

*   Were you able to maintain the same level of concentration throughout the entire examination?

*   Did you have adequate time to complete the examination?

- Did you effectively incorporate test taking strategies?

- Did you misinterpret or fail to identify what selected questions were asking?

- Did the questions that were answered incorrectly exhibit any similar characteristics?

- Did you make any careless mistakes?

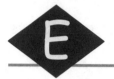

Exercise: Physical Therapist Assistant Examination

Each candidate will have a maximum of three hours to complete the 150 question examination. Candidates should attempt to take the examination in a single designated three hour period. By completing the examination in this fashion, candidates can make the sample examination more realistic, and therefore will be able to gather more accurate information on their performance.

Attempt to identify the best answer to each question. After completing the examination, utilize the answer key located at the conclusion of the exercise to determine the number of questions answered correctly. Record your score for the examination on the performance analysis summary sheet located in the Appendix. The criterion-referenced passing score for this sample examination is 112. Therefore a score of 112 or more would be a passing score and a score of less than 112 would be a failing score.

Candidate performance on the sample examination should be used only as a method to assess strengths and weaknesses and should not be utilized as a predictor of actual examination performance. Any similarity in the questions contained within the sample examination and a question on any version of the Physical Therapist Assistant Examination is purely coincidental.

Sample Physical Therapist Assistant Examination

1. After observing a patient during an exercise session, a physical therapist assistant concludes that the patient commonly uses the Valsalva maneuver. Which activity would have the greatest probability of producing the Valsalva maneuver?

    1. lifting a 40 lb. package from the floor to a counter at waist level
    2. walking at 4 mph on a treadmill
    3. stationary cycling at 80 revolutions per minute
    4. using an upper extremity ergometer at 40 revolutions per minute

2. A physical therapist assistant employed in an acute care hospital works with a patient on bed mobility activities. The therapist would like to incorporate a strengthening activity for the hip extensors that will improve the patient's ability to independently reposition in bed, however the patient does not have adequate strength to perform bridging. The most appropriate exercise activity is:

    1. anterior pelvic tilts
    2. heel slides
    3. straight leg raises
    4. isometric gluteal sets

3. A physical therapist assistant prepares to perform manual vibration as part of a plan of care for a patient with chronic obstructive pulmonary disease. The most appropriate time to administer the technique is after a:

    1. normal inspiration
    2. deep inspiration
    3. normal expiration
    4. deep expiration

4. A physical therapist assistant obtains a baseline value for inspiratory capacity using an incentive spirometer as part of a preoperative session. Which measurement would be the most consistent with the expected normal value?

    1. 1,000 mL
    2. 3,000 mL
    3. 5,000 mL
    4. 7,000 mL

5. A physical therapist assistant instructs a patient status post abdominal surgery how to use an incentive spirometer in order to prevent the occurrence of pulmonary complications. The most appropriate frequency for the patient to use the incentive spirometer is:

1. once each ten minutes
2. once every two hours
3. twice per day
4. once per day

6. A physical therapist assistant employed in an outpatient private practice treats a patient diagnosed with spondylolisthesis. Which of the following scenarios would be most consistent with the medical diagnosis?

1. a 13-year-old female gymnast with no significant medical history
2. a 17-year-old female tennis player with a 15 degree lateral curvature of the spine
3. a 28-year-old male machinist with a history of recurrent lower back pain
4. a 67-year-old male with a previous diagnosis of ankylosing spondylitis

7. A 66-year-old male rehabilitating from a shoulder injury uses an upper body ergometer as part of a rehabilitation program. The physical therapist assistant would like the patient to use the ergometer at 40 revolutions per minute for 12 minutes. The patient maintains an active lifestyle despite the implantation of a fixed rate pacemaker six years ago. The most appropriate method to monitor the intensity of exercise during the session is:

1. heart rate
2. blood pressure
3. respiration rate
4. rating of perceived exertion

8. A physical therapist assistant reviews the medical record of a patient recently diagnosed with peripheral vascular disease. A note in the medical record indicates that the patient's ankle-brachial index (ABI) was within normal limits. The value most consistent with this measure is:

1. .5
2. .7
3. 1.0
4. 1.3

9. A patient with a 40 degree limitation in right shoulder flexion and a 35 degree limitation in lateral rotation is unable to perform a number of activities of daily living. Which activity would be the most difficult for the patient using the right upper extremity?

    1. tucking in shirt
    2. combing hair
    3. eating
    4. washing the left shoulder

10. A patient rehabilitating from a CVA exhibits a flexor synergy pattern in the upper extremity. The strongest component of the flexor synergy pattern is:

    1. shoulder lateral rotation
    2. forearm supination
    3. elbow flexion
    4. scapular elevation

11. A patient being treated in an outpatient orthopedic clinic begins to demonstrate signs and symptoms of CVA including unilateral weakness, unexplained dizziness, and loss of vision. Recognizing the symptoms of a CVA, the physical therapist assistant begins to administer first aid. Which of the following would not be considered appropriate first aid management?

    1. monitor the airway, breathing and circulation
    2. remove mucus from the mouth with a piece of cloth wrapped around a finger
    3. lay the patient down and slightly elevate the legs
    4. immediately contact medical assistance

12. A physical therapist assistant working in a special care unit notices a tiny air bubble in a peripheral IV line. The therapist's most immediate response should be to:

    1. turn off the IV
    2. remove the IV
    3. reposition the peripheral IV line
    4. continue with the present treatment

13. A physical therapist assistant prepares a presentation on proper body mechanics for a group of 100 autoworkers. Which of the following media would be most effective to maximize learning during the presentation?

    1. lecture, handouts
    2. lecture, charts, statistics
    3. lecture, handouts, demonstration
    4. lecture, statistics

14. A physical therapist assistant performs a number of upper extremity goniometric measurements on a patient rehabilitating from injuries sustained in a motor vehicle accident. Which of the following measurements would not be conducted with the patient in supine?

    1. shoulder flexion
    2. wrist flexion
    3. hip flexion
    4. hip abduction

The following information should be used to answer questions 15 and 16:

A physical therapist assistant treats a 22-year-old female athlete who sustained an ankle sprain three days ago playing soccer. The patient is currently full weight bearing, however walks with an antalgic gait. In order to assess the ligamentous integrity of the ankle, the therapist prepares to administer the anterior drawer test. The therapist positions the patient in supine and stabilizes the tibia and fibula.

15. The most appropriate method for performing the anterior drawer test is:

    1. maintain the foot in neutral and draw the talus forward
    2. maintain the foot in 20 degrees of plantar flexion and draw the talus forward
    3. maintain the foot in neutral and draw the calcaneus forward
    4. maintain the foot in 20 degrees of plantar flexion and draw the calcaneus forward

16. A positive anterior drawer test would be, at the very least, indicative of:

    1. disruption to the anterior talofibular ligament
    2. disruption to the calcaneofibular ligament
    3. disruption to the anterior talofibular ligament and calcaneofibular ligament
    4. disruption of the anterior talofibular ligament, calcaneofibular ligament, and deltoid ligament

17. A 66-year-old female is referred to physical therapy with rheumatoid arthritis. During treatment the physical therapist assistant notes increased flexion at the proximal interphalangeal joints and hyperextension at the distal interphalangeal joints. This deformity is commonly termed:

    1. boutonniere deformity
    2. mallet finger
    3. swan neck deformity
    4. ulnar drift

18. A physical therapist assistant discusses the importance of proper nutrition with a patient diagnosed with congestive heart failure. Which of the following substances would be most restricted in this patient's diet?

    1. cholesterol
    2. potassium
    3. sodium
    4. triglycerides

19. A physical therapist assistant uses a S.O.A.P. note format for his daily documentation. Which of the following would not be found in the assessment section of a S.O.A.P. note?

    1. short and long-term goals
    2. discussion of a patient's progress in therapy
    3. patient's equipment needs and equipment ordered
    4. patient's rehabilitation potential

20. Physical therapist assistants use a wide variety of measurement methods in their daily documentation. Which of the following measurement methods would not be considered objective?

    1. duration of attention
    2. goniometric measurements
    3. rating on a perceived exertion scale
    4. time required to perform a selected activity

21. Physical therapist assistants often communicate with patients using open-ended questions. Which of the following questions would not be considered open-ended?

    1. What makes your pain better?
    2. Is your back more painful at night?
    3. How does exercise effect your back?
    4. Describe your activities in a typical day?

22. A patient is scheduled to undergo a transtibial amputation secondary to poor healing of an ulcer on his left foot. In addition, the patient is two months status post right knee replacement due to osteoarthritis. Given the patient's past and current medical history, the physical therapist assistant can expect which of the following tasks to be the most difficult for the patient following the amputation?

    1. rolling from supine to sidelying
    2. moving from sitting to supine
    3. moving from sitting to standing
    4. ambulating in the parallel bars

23. A physical therapist assistant wears sterile protective clothing while treating a patient. Which area of the protective clothing would be considered non-sterile even before coming in contact with a non-sterile object?

    1. gloves
    2. sleeves of the gown
    3. front of the gown above waist level
    4. front of the gown below waist level

24. A physical therapist assistant positions a patient in prone in preparation for manual muscle testing. When testing the medial hamstrings the therapist should apply resistance against the:

    1. leg; distal to the ankle in the direction of knee extension
    2. leg; distal to the ankle in the direction of knee flexion
    3. leg; proximal to the ankle in the direction of knee extension
    4. leg; proximal to the ankle in the direction of knee flexion

25. A patient two days status post transfemoral amputation demonstrates decreased strength and generalized deconditioning. Which of the following positions should be utilized when wrapping the patient's residual limb?

    1. sidelying
    2. standing
    3. supine
    4. prone

26. A patient two days status post transtibial amputation complains of phantom sensation. Which of the following treatment options would be inappropriate?

    1. tell the patient to leave the residual limb exposed to the air at all times
    2. discuss the option of a temporary prosthesis with the patient's physician
    3. begin residual limb wrapping
    4. teach the patient to tap and massage the residual limb

27. A physical therapist assistant transports a patient with multiple sclerosis to the gym for her treatment session. The patient is wheelchair dependent and uses a urinary catheter. When transporting the patient, the most appropriate location to secure the collection bag is:

    1. in the patient's lap
    2. on the patient's lower abdomen
    3. on the wheelchair armrest
    4. on the wheelchair cross brace beneath the seat

28. A physical therapist assistant examines a patient with multiple sclerosis The patient has poor to fair strength in her legs, good arm strength, and moderate truncal ataxia. The safest means for the patient to ambulate in her home would be:

    1. with a single point cane
    2. with a walker
    3. while holding onto furniture or walls
    4. with axillary crutches

29. A physical therapist assistant treats a patient diagnosed with cerebellar degeneration. Which of the following signs/symptoms is not characteristic of cerebellar degeneration?

   1. limb ataxia
   2. nystagmus
   3. wide base of support when ambulating
   4. hypertonia

30. A male physical therapist assistant treats a 16-year-old female with low back pain. During the treatment session the patient makes several sexually suggestive remarks. The therapist ignores the remarks, but the patient reiterates them during the next treatment session. The most appropriate therapist action is to:

   1. continue to ignore the patient's remarks
   2. explain to the patient that her remarks are offensive
   3. document the patient's behavior in the medical record
   4. contact the supervising physical therapist

31. A physical therapist assistant provides preoperative instruction for a patient scheduled for anterior cruciate ligament reconstructive surgery. During the treatment session, the patient expresses to the therapist a sincere fear of dying during surgery. The therapist's most appropriate response would be:

   1. This surgery is done many times every day.
   2. I have never had a patient of mine die yet.
   3. Surgery can be a very frightening thought.
   4. You will be back to athletics before you know it.

32. A physical therapist reads in the medical record that a patient experiences frequent premature ventricular contractions. Which of the following does not precipitate PVCs?

   1. anxiety
   2. tobacco
   3. alcohol
   4. sodium

33. A physical therapist assistant instructs a patient in ambulation activities using axillary crutches. What two points of control should be used when guarding the patient?

1. the patient's thorax and hip
2. the patient's shoulder and hip
3. the patient's shoulder and thorax
4. the patient's elbow and hip

34. A physical therapist assistant assesses the functional strength of a patient's hip extensors while observing a patient move from standing to sitting. What type of contraction occurs in the hip extensors during this activity?

1. concentric
2. eccentric
3. isometric
4. isotonic

35. A patient with cardiopulmonary pathology is referred to physical therapy. The physical therapist assistant documents the following clinical signs: pallor, cyanosis, and skin coolness. These clinical signs are most consistent with:

1. cor pulmonale
2. anemia
3. atelectasis
4. diaphoresis

36. A physical therapist assistant treats a 36-year-old male status post knee surgery. The therapist performs goniometric measurements to quantify the extent of the patient's extension lag. Which of the following would not provide a plausible rationale for the extension lag?

1. muscle weakness
2. bony obstruction
3. inhibition by pain
4. patient apprehension

37. A physical therapist assistant listens to the lung sounds of a 56-year-old male with chronic bronchitis. The patient was admitted to the hospital two days ago after complaining of shortness of breath and difficulty breathing. While performing auscultation the therapist identifies distinct lung sounds with a relatively high constant pitch during exhalation. This type of sound is most consistent with:

1. crackles
2. rales
3. rhonchi
4. wheezes

38. A physical therapist assistant examines a patient's lower extremity strength. In order to accurately assess the gluteus medius, the therapist should position the patient in:

1. prone
2. sidelying
3. sitting
4. supine

39. A physical therapist assistant is a member of an interdisciplinary team in a rehabilitation center. One of the patients on the pediatric unit is a 5-year-old boy who sustained a head injury and multiple fractures in a motor vehicle accident. The patient is scheduled to be treated by the team, but there is no information in the medical chart which specifies the patient's weight bearing status. Which member of the interdisciplinary team would be responsible for determining the patient's weight bearing status?

1. physical therapist
2. occupational therapist
3. speech therapist
4. physician

40. A patient files suit against a physical therapist assistant claiming that he was injured as a result of a specific intervention. In legal proceedings, which of the following would have the most impact on what actually happened at the time of the alleged negligent act?

1. the patient's recollections
2. the physical therapist assistant's recollections
3. the referring physician's examination
4. the physical therapist assistant's daily documentation

41. A physical therapist assistant prepares to perform a Lachman test on a patient with a suspected anterior cruciate ligament injury. Why is the Lachman test considered to be more accurate than the anterior drawer test?

1. hand placement is more difficult in the anterior drawer test
2. the anterior joint capsule is more lax in the anterior drawer test
3. the hamstrings pull in direct opposition to the anterior drawer test and often prevent anterior translation of the tibia on the femur
4. the shape of the menisci allow greater anterior tibial translation in a position emphasizing knee flexion

42. A physical therapist assistant instructs a patient rehabilitating from a lower extremity injury to descend stairs using axillary crutches. Assuming the patient is partial weight bearing, which sequence is the most appropriate?

1. crutches, involved leg, uninvolved leg
2. crutches, uninvolved leg, involved leg
3. uninvolved leg, crutches, involved leg
4. involved leg, crutches, uninvolved leg

43. A physical therapist assistant discusses potential functional outcomes for patients after complete spinal cord injuries. Which spinal cord injury level would provide a patient with the best opportunity to functionally ambulate?

1. C7
2. T1
3. T6
4. L1

44. A physical therapy clinic purchases a pelvic traction unit. Which of the following conditions is not a relative contraindication for pelvic traction?

1. pregnancy
2. herniated nucleus pulposus with disc protrusion
3. osteoporosis
4. hiatal hernia

45. A physical therapist assistant stimulates an innervated muscle at its motor point with a brief direct current. Which of the following types of muscular response would be expected?

    1. a tetanic response to continuous current stimulation
    2. a brisk contraction followed by a rapid relaxation
    3. a brisk contraction followed by a sluggish relaxation
    4. there will be no muscular response

46. A physical therapist assistant discusses total hip replacement precautions with a patient following surgery. Which statement would not be considered good advice?

    1. sit in low chairs
    2. do not cross your legs
    3. do not bend down to pick up objects off the floor
    4. keep a pillow between your legs while sleeping

47. A physical therapist assistant commonly uses superficial and deep heat to increase blood flow to facilitate tissue healing. Which type of pharmacological agent would have an antagonistic effect on the desired objective?

    1. anti-inflammatory steroids
    2. nonsteroidal anti-inflammatory drugs
    3. peripheral vasodilators
    4. systemic vasoconstrictors

48. When performing range of motion exercises with a patient who sustained a traumatic brain injury, a physical therapist assistant notes that the patient lacks full elbow extension and classifies the end-feel as hard. The most likely cause is:

    1. heterotopic ossification
    2. spasticity of the biceps
    3. anterior capsular tightness
    4. triceps weakness

49. A physical therapist assistant interviews a 21-year-old football player referred to physical therapy after sustaining a grade II acromioclavicular sprain. Which of the following patient descriptions best describes the injury mechanism associated with an acromioclavicular sprain?

 1. "I was being tackled and landed directly on my shoulder."
 2. "I fell with my arm extended and another player fell on top of me."
 3. "My arm was hit with a helmet while I was throwing the ball."
 4. "My arm was stepped on while I was lying on the ground."

50. A physical therapist and a physical therapist assistant employed in an acute care hospital are responsible for providing weekend therapy coverage. After examining the patient treatment list, the therapists attempt to develop an action plan. Which of the following activities would be the least appropriate for the physical therapist assistant?

 1. instruct a patient in prosthetic donning and doffing
 2. assist a patient with ambulation activities
 3. examine a patient referred to physical therapy for instruction in a home exercise program
 4. perform goniometric measurements on a patient one day status post anterior cruciate ligament reconstruction

51. A physical therapist assistant instructs a patient diagnosed with peroneal tendonitis in a home exercise program. As part of the program the therapist would like the patient to apply superficial heat to the injured area before beginning a stretching exercise. Which of the following modalities would be the most effective for the patient to incorporate into the program?

 1. diathermy
 2. paraffin
 3. pulsed ultrasound
 4. warm water bath

52. A physical therapist assistant records the following entry in a patient's medical record: active right knee flexion 20-70 degrees. Based on the medical record, which of the following statements is not accurate?

 1. The patient has 50 degrees of available range of motion in the right knee.
 2. The patient can flex the right knee to 70 degrees.
 3. The patient's knee is hypermobile.
 4. The patient has limited right knee range of motion.

53. A physical therapist assistant performs a home assessment for a patient preparing for discharge from a rehabilitation hospital. The patient sustained an incomplete spinal cord injury 11 weeks ago and currently uses a wheelchair for all mobility. Which of the following is likely to be the most significant architectural barrier for the patient?

   1. hardwood floors
   2. an entrance ramp (six inches of ramp for every one inch of step height)
   3. one quarter inch thresholds at each door
   4. pedestal type sinks

54. A physical therapist assistant participates in a study that examines the effect of goniometer size on the reliability of passive shoulder joint measurements. The study concludes that goniometric passive measurements of shoulder range of motion can be highly reliable when taken by a single therapist regardless of the size of the goniometer. This study demonstrates the use of:

   1. interrater reliability
   2. intrarater reliability
   3. interrater validity
   4. intrarater validity

55. A patient with a confirmed posterior cruciate ligament tear is able to return to full dynamic activities following rehabilitation. Which of the following does not serve as a secondary restraint to the posterior cruciate ligament?

   1. iliotibial band
   2. popliteus tendon
   3. lateral collateral ligament
   4. medial collateral ligament

56. A physical therapist assistant transports a patient with a traumatic brain injury to the physical therapy gym. Each day after arriving in the gym, the patient asks the therapist, "Where am I?" Recognizing the patient has short-term memory loss, the therapist's most appropriate response should be:

   1. You know where you are.
   2. You are in the same place you were yesterday at this time.
   3. You are in the physical therapy gym for your treatment session.
   4. You are in the hospital because of your injury.

57. A physical therapist assistant presents an inservice on ergonomics for administrative personnel. As part of the presentation, the therapist discusses positioning when seated at a computer terminal. Which of the following recommendations would be most helpful?

    1. position your thighs parallel with the floor
    2. position your knees one inch above your hips
    3. position your knees two inches above your hips
    4. position your knees one inch below your hips

58. An eight-year-old female with a 25 degree scoliotic curve is fitted for a Milwaukee brace. The brace will likely be worn until:

    1. the scoliotic curve does not increase within a one year period
    2. the patient resumes all recreational and athletic activities
    3. the patient is pain free for six months
    4. spinal growth ceases

59. A physical therapist assistant works with a patient diagnosed with anterior compartment syndrome. The patient presents with an inability to dorsiflex the foot and a mild sensory disturbance between the first and second toes. The nerve most likely involved is the:

    1. deep peroneal nerve
    2. medial plantar nerve
    3. tibial nerve
    4. lateral plantar nerve

60. A physical therapist assistant participates in a community fitness program by conducting anthropometric measurements designed to determine percent body fat. Which site is not typically utilized when measuring skinfolds?

    1. iliac crest
    2. subscapular
    3. triceps
    4. lateral calf

61. A physical therapist assistant treats a patient diagnosed with temporomandibular joint dysfunction. The therapist believes the patient's clinical presentation is consistent with an anterior disk dislocation that does not reduce during joint translation. The most characteristic finding with this type of condition is:

1. excessive crepitation during mouth opening and closing
2. restricted mouth opening
3. loud click or pop during mouth opening
4. constant pain

62. A physical therapist assistant works with a 38-year-old female diagnosed with rheumatoid arthritis. The patient presents with muscle weakness, joint stiffness, and limited motion. The patient is extremely warm to the touch over involved joints and has moderate swelling. Which of the following would not be a component of the patient's current care plan?

1. modalities
2. immobilization in a splint
3. active stretching exercises
4. muscle setting exercises

63. A physical therapist assistant completes a manual muscle test of the flexor digitorum brevis. In order to accurately assess the strength of the muscle, the therapist should apply pressure against the:

1. dorsal surface of the middle phalanx of the four toes in the direction of extension
2. plantar surface of the middle phalanx of the four toes in the direction of extension
3. dorsal surface of the distal phalanx of the four toes in the direction of extension
4. plantar surface of the distal phalanx of the four toes in the direction of extension

64. A patient with complete tetraplegia at the C5 level is referred to a rehabilitation hospital for eight weeks of therapy. Which of the following is not a realistic goal for the patient?

1. able to complete lower extremity self-stretching in bed independently
2. able to eat independently with adaptive equipment
3. able to propel a manual wheelchair 15 feet on level surfaces independently
4. able to direct a caretaker to perform a car transfer

65. A physical therapist assistant is required to transfer a 250 lb. dependent patient from a mat table to a wheelchair. The therapist is concerned about her ability to independently transfer the patient, but is unable to locate another staff member to offer assistance. The most appropriate action would be to:

    1. instruct the patient to take a more active role in the transfer
    2. attempt to complete the transfer independently, but stop immediately if body mechanics are compromised
    3. inform the nursing staff to complete the transfer
    4. wait until another staff member is available to assist with the transfer

66. A physical therapist assistant interviews a patient referred to physical therapy diagnosed with carpal tunnel syndrome. Which question would be considered open-ended?

    1. Do you have difficulty operating a keyboard?
    2. Do you have pain with repetitive motion?
    3. How many breaks do you take during an eight hour shift?
    4. How well are you able to complete assigned activities?

67. A physical therapist assistant assesses a patient's shoulder lateral rotation in supine. When completing a goniometric measurement, the therapist should position the stationary arm of the goniometer:

    1. perpendicular to the floor
    2. parallel with the inferior midline of the humerus
    3. parallel with the olecranon process
    4. parallel with the lateral midline of the humerus

68. A patient sustains a traction injury to the brachial plexus in a motor vehicle accident and has resultant C5 and C6 nerve root involvement. Which of the following muscles would be most affected by the injury?

    1. flexor carpi ulnaris
    2. levator scapulae
    3. pectoralis minor
    4. pectoralis major

69. A physical therapist assistant discusses the importance of proper skin care with a patient and his family. Which of the following sites is least likely to develop a pressure ulcer in a wheelchair dependent patient?

    1. scapula
    2. ischium
    3. heel
    4. elbow

70. A physical therapist assistant assesses a patient's lower extremity deep tendon reflexes using a reflex hammer. Which of the following reflexes would provide the therapist with the most information on the L3-L4 spinal level?

    1. patellar reflex
    2. lateral hamstrings reflex
    3. posterior tibial reflex
    4. Achilles reflex

71. A physical therapist assistant treats a patient with a traumatic head injury. The patient is currently classified as confused-agitated on the Rancho Los Amigos Level of Cognitive Functioning Scale. Which of the following guidelines would be the least beneficial when developing the treatment program?

    1. The therapist should emphasize previously learned skills and avoid teaching only new skills.
    2. The therapist should maintain a calm and focused affect.
    3. The therapist should concentrate on one specific activity for each treatment session.
    4. The therapist should schedule the patient at the same time and same place each day.

72. A physical therapist assistant presents an inservice entitled "Preventing Pressure Ulcers" to a group of physical therapy aides. As part of the inservice the therapist identifies risk factors associated with the development of pressure ulcers. Which of the following would not be considered a significant risk factor?

    1. nutritional deficiencies
    2. incontinence
    3. psychological stress and depression
    4. vocational dysfunction

73. A patient sustains a chemical burn on the cubital area of the elbow. Which position would be the most appropriate for splinting of the involved upper extremity?

    1. elbow flexion and forearm pronation
    2. elbow flexion and forearm supination
    3. elbow extension and forearm pronation
    4. elbow extension and forearm supination

74. A patient with a C7 nerve root injury is treated in physical therapy. Which of the following objective findings would be most indicative of C7 involvement?

    1. paresthesias over the little finger
    2. weak triceps and wrist flexor muscles
    3. paresthesias over the thumb
    4. weak biceps and supinator muscles

75. A physical therapist assistant employed in a skilled nursing facility frequently treats cognitively impaired elderly patients. Which of the following guidelines is not recommended when working with this particular population?

    1. encourage the use of hands on treatment
    2. explain frequently, consistently, and repetitively when necessary
    3. change the patient's environment and staff frequently
    4. simplify commands and label items for easy recognition

76. Members of a health promotion task force design a program that will annually screen individuals in selected retirement communities for osteoporosis. Which screening tool would be the most cost effective and reliable to incorporate as part of the screening program?

    1. physical activity survey
    2. dietary analysis
    3. measuring height
    4. urinalysis screening

77. A physical therapist assistant prepares a patient for prosthetic training. Which of the following amputations would require the highest energy expenditure when using the appropriate prosthesis?

    1. bilateral transtibial amputations
    2. unilateral transtibial amputation
    3. unilateral transfemoral amputation
    4. Syme's amputation

78. A physical therapist assistant returns to work after a brief luncheon meeting and finds a number of items that require her immediate attention. Which of the following items should be given the highest priority?

    1. an unattended patient exercising in the gym
    2. a scheduled patient that has been waiting for 15 minutes
    3. a laboratory test report that has not been reviewed
    4. a patient record that has not been completed

79. A physical therapist assistant utilizes the results of a symptom-limited exercise treadmill test to determine the intensity of exercise for a patient who previously sustained a cardiac event. Which of the following guidelines would be the most appropriate when determining an appropriate exercise intensity for the patient?

    1. 20 percent of the maximal heart rate obtained on the treadmill test
    2. 40 percent of the maximal heart rate obtained on the treadmill test
    3. 60 percent of the maximal heart rate obtained on the treadmill test
    4. 80 percent of the maximal heart rate obtained on the treadmill test

80. A physical therapist assistant instructs a patient to complete a biceps strengthening exercise using a fifteen pound dumbbell in standing. The exercise requires the patient to maximally flex the elbow twelve times without moving the trunk. While observing the patient perform the exercise, it becomes apparent that the patient is unable to maintain the trunk in a stationary position. Which of the following would be the most appropriate action to modify the exercise?

    1. decrease the number of repetitions to six
    2. decrease the dumbbell weight to ten pounds
    3. instruct the patient to perform the exercise while sitting on a stool
    4. no modification is necessary

81. A physical therapist assistant treats a patient diagnosed with chronic arterial insufficiency. Assuming the patient does not demonstrate pain at rest, which of the following treatment techniques would be contraindicated for the patient?

    1. ambulation with an assistive device
    2. patient education regarding proper skin care
    3. stationary cycling
    4. ankle pumps with legs elevated

82. A physical therapist assistant treats a patient diagnosed with Guillain-Barre syndrome. All of the following are signs or symptoms associated with this syndrome except:

    1. difficulty breathing
    2. areflexia
    3. weakness
    4. absent sensation

83. A physical therapist assistant completes a daily progress note utilizing a S.O.A.P. format. Which of the following entries would not belong in the objective section?

    1. will receive continuous ultrasound to the right anterior shoulder at 1.5 W/cm^2 for 5 minutes
    2. incision on the left anterior forearm covered with steri-strips
    3. left lower extremity range of motion within normal limits
    4. tenderness to palpation in L1-L2 region

84. A physical therapist assistant treats a patient referred to physical therapy after being diagnosed with arteriosclerosis obliterans. The therapist begins a walking program with the patient on a treadmill. After two minutes of walking at 1.0 mile per hour the patient reports significant cramping and pain in her lower legs. The most appropriate therapist action is to:

    1. encourage the patient to walk through the pain until it becomes unbearable
    2. decrease the treadmill speed by one-half mile per hour and instruct the patient to continue walking
    3. allow the patient to rest and resume walking when the pain subsides
    4. discontinue walking and select an alternate exercise

85. A 23-year-old male sustains serious burns to over 40% of his body in a house fire. The burns range from superficial partial-thickness to full-thickness and encompass the majority of the patient's lower extremities. The most appropriate therapeutic position for the patient is:

1. supine with the knees extended and the toes pointing toward the ceiling
2. prone with a pillow placed on the dorsum of the foot and ankle
3. sidelying with the hip and knees slightly flexed with pillows between the legs
4. hooklying with a pillow placed between the knees

86. A physical therapist assistant treats a patient with Parkinson's disease. The patient has trouble initiating movement and is unable to ambulate independently. The patient reports that he has fallen on three separate occasions within the last two months while attempting to ambulate. Which assistive device would be the most appropriate for the patient?

1. rolling walker
2. walker
3. axillary crutches
4. small base quad cane

87. A physical therapist assistant positions a patient in prone and passively flexes his knee. As the knee flexes, the patient's hip on the same side also begins to flex. This clinical finding is most indicative of a:

1. tight iliopsoas
2. tight rectus femoris
3. tight tensor fasciae latae
4. tight hamstrings

88. A physical therapist assistant measures the hip range of motion of a patient with excessive anteversion. Which of the following clinical findings would be the most common?

1. increased hip lateral rotation and decreased medial rotation
2. increased hip medial rotation and decreased lateral rotation
3. increased hip abduction and decreased adduction
4. increased hip flexion and decreased extension

89. A physical therapist assistant obtains measurements of 73 degrees and 75 degrees on two successive goniometric measurements of shoulder medial rotation. The ability to measure the range of motion consistently is primarily a function of:

   1. biological variation
   2. standard deviation
   3. reliability
   4. validity

90. A patient has diminished calf sensation and an absent Achilles reflex on the right lower extremity. The patient had earlier communicated to the physical therapist assistant that she experienced difficulty controlling her bowel movements. The neurologic level of most concern is:

   1. L2
   2. L4
   3. L5
   4. S2

91. A patient with hemiplegia ambulates with an ankle-foot orthosis. The physical therapist assistant notes that the patient's involved foot frequently drags along the floor throughout swing phase. To treat this problem most effectively, the therapist should emphasize increasing the strength of the:

   1. quadriceps
   2. iliopsoas
   3. gluteus medius
   4. hamstrings

92. Which of the following techniques will most effectively increase a patient's hip stability?

   1. lower trunk rotation in the hooklying position
   2. bridging
   3. assisted hip and knee flexion in supine
   4. hip abduction and adduction in the hooklying position

93. A physical therapist assistant completes a posture screening and a gross range of motion assessment on a patient referred to therapy with patella tendonitis. The therapist determines that the patient has extremely limited lower extremity flexibility, most notably in the hip flexors. What common structural condition is often associated with tight hip flexors?

1. scoliosis
2. kyphosis
3. lordosis
4. spondylosis

94. A physical therapist assistant determines that a patient has a one half inch leg length discrepancy. The therapist suspects the patient's leg length discrepancy may be due to tibial shortening. The most appropriate measurement to confirm the therapist's suspicions is from the:

1. anterior superior iliac spine to the medial malleolus
2. iliac crest to the lateral malleolus
3. medial knee joint line to the medial malleolus
4. lateral knee joint line to the medial malleolus

95. A physical therapist assistant conducts a goniometric assessment of a patient's upper extremities. Which of the following values is most indicative of normal passive glenohumeral abduction?

1. 50 degrees
2. 116 degrees
3. 155 degrees
4. 178 degrees

96. A physical therapist assistant reviews the results of an assessment performed on a child with cerebral palsy. The record indicates that the child is able to hop on a single foot 3-5 times, throw a ball eight feet, jump forward two feet, and cut with scissors. The child is not able to gallop, skip, or button his shirt. Based on the child's gross and fine motor skills, the child is developmentally functioning at a:

1. 2 year-old level
2. 3-4 year-old level
3. 5-7 year-old level
4. 9-10 year old level

97. While preparing a sterile field for wound debridement, a physical therapist assistant accidentally places a nonsterile object on the sterile base. The most appropriate action is to:

1. remove the nonsterile object from the sterile base and continue with treatment
2. continue with treatment, however be sure no other supplies come in contact with the nonsterile object
3. remove all of the items to be used from the sterile base and replace them with similar items that are sterile
4. discard the entire sterile field and establish a new sterile field

98. A patient with a fractured right humerus receives physical therapy services. The therapist determines goniometrically that the patient can actively flex his right shoulder to 178 degrees. Which of the following entries would be the most appropriate to illustrate the physical therapist assistant's findings?

1. right shoulder flexion range of motion is 0-178 degrees
2. right shoulder range of motion is within normal limits
3. right shoulder flexion active range of motion to 178 degrees
4. right shoulder active range of motion to 178 degrees

99. A physical therapist assistant works with a patient placed in isolation. The therapist is required to wear a mask while treating the patient, but is not required to wear gloves or a gown. This type of isolation is best termed:

1. strict isolation
2. contact isolation
3. respiratory isolation
4. blood/body fluid precautions

100. A physical therapist assistant engages in therapeutic play with a 10 month old infant diagnosed with developmental delay. The medical record indicates the child is functioning at a six to seven month old level. Which activity would the child likely be able to perform?

1. pulls to stand from half-kneel position
2. creeps on hands and knees
3. cruises along furniture
4. assumes sitting position independently

101. A patient, who is status post CVA and presents with Wernicke's aphasia, is learning how to perform a sit to stand transfer. Which option would be least effective to incorporate into the teaching session?

    1. using a mirror for visual feedback
    2. providing detailed instructions
    3. using repetition
    4. demonstrating

102. A patient status post total hip replacement is referred to physical therapy for gait training. The patient has not been weight bearing on the involved lower extremity since surgery and appears to be somewhat anxious. The most appropriate setting to begin ambulation activities is:

    1. in the parallel bars
    2. in the parallel bars with a rolling walker
    3. in the physical therapy gym with a straight cane
    4. in the physical therapy gym with a walker

103. A patient involved in a motor vehicle accident sustains a Colles' fracture and an intertrochanteric hip fracture. The patient has been cleared for toe-touch weight bearing by the physician. Which assistive device would be the most appropriate for the patient?

    1. straight cane
    2. axillary crutches
    3. rolling walker
    4. walker with a platform attachment

104. A physical therapist assistant instructs a 55-year-old patient with bilateral lower extremity paralysis to transfer from a wheelchair to a mat table. The patient has normal upper extremity strength and has no other known medical problems. The most appropriate transfer technique is a:

    1. dependent standing pivot
    2. sliding board transfer
    3. two person carry
    4. hydraulic lift

105. A physical therapist assistant instructs a patient to make a fist. The patient can make a fist, but is unable to flex the distal phalanx of his ring finger. This clinical finding can best be explained by:

1. a ruptured flexor carpi radialis tendon
2. a ruptured flexor digitorum superficialis tendon
3. a ruptured flexor digitorum profundus tendon
4. a ruptured extensor digitorum communis tendon

106. A nine month old infant with cerebral palsy is unable to roll from prone to supine. This developmental activity typically occurs by:

1. 3 months
2. 5 months
3. 7 months
4. 9 months

The following information should be used to answer questions 107 and 108:

A male patient with complete T10 paraplegia accompanies a physical therapist assistant and occupational therapist on a home visit prior to being discharged from a rehabilitation hospital. The patient has been in the hospital for 12 weeks and has had an unremarkable recovery. The patient resides alone in a two bedroom ranch, however has numerous family in the area who will be able to periodically assist him. As part of the home visit the therapists examine accessibility.

107. Which item would be most problematic for the patient?

1. an outdoor ramp that is 36 inches wide
2. an outdoor ramp with an 8.3% grade
3. a bathroom sink with 24 inches of clearance under the sink
4. a doorway that is 32 inches wide

108. Based on the patient's diagnosis and his living situation, the patient would most likely:

1. require regular assistance from a home health aide for activities of daily living
2. utilize a wheelchair for functional mobility
3. utilize orthotics and a walker for household and community ambulation
4. be unable to safely return to his home

109. A physical therapist assistant attempts to measure a patient's elbow flexion range of motion. While conducting the measurement, the therapist should stabilize the:

1. radius and ulna
2. thorax
3. proximal humerus
4. distal humerus

110. A physical therapist assistant instructs a patient rehabilitating from a transfemoral amputation on the importance of positioning. Which of the following positions would leave the patient most susceptible to a lower extremity contracture?

1. prone lying
2. supine with the residual limb elevated on a pillow
3. supine
4. sidelying

111. A physical therapist assistant observes a patient ambulating with axillary crutches. The patient uses the crutches to support her weight as she advances her weight bearing lower extremity. This description best describes a:

1. two-point gait pattern
2. three-point gait pattern
3. four-point gait pattern
4. swing-through

112. A physical therapist assistant fits a patient for axillary crutches in preparation for gait training. Which of the following statements regarding axillary crutches is not accurate?

1. Axillary crutches require good standing balance.
2. Axillary crutches offer limited support due to a small base of support.
3. Axillary crutches are less stable than a walker.
4. Functional strength of the upper extremities is required for most gait patterns.

113. A physical therapist assistant prepares a whirlpool for a patient with cardiovascular disease. Which of the following water temperatures would be inappropriate for the patient?

    1. 30 degrees Celsius
    2. 33 degrees Celsius
    3. 36 degrees Celsius
    4. 40 degrees Celsius

114. A physical therapist assistant prepares to use cryotherapy on a patient's knee following an exercise session. Which of the following is not a precaution when using cryotherapy?

    1. Raynaud's phenomenon
    2. cold intolerance
    3. cryoglobinemia
    4. epiphyseal areas in children

115. A physical therapist assistant instructs a patient how to monitor her pulse rate using the radial artery. To accurately locate the radial pulse, the patient should palpate:

    1. on the dorsal surface of the wrist, just lateral to the styloid process of the radius
    2. on the dorsal surface of the wrist, just medial to the styloid process of the radius
    3. on the volar surface of the wrist, just lateral to the styloid process of the radius
    4. on the volar surface of the wrist, just medial to the styloid process of the radius

116. A physical therapist assistant instructs a patient to perform a series of exercises at home. As part of the program, the therapist provides specific instructions regarding the frequency and duration of each exercise. To maximize the patient's understanding and compliance with the exercise program, the therapist should:

    1. demonstrate each exercise
    2. emphasize the importance of selected exercises
    3. provide written instructions, in addition to the oral instructions
    4. demonstrate each exercise and provide written instructions

117. A physical therapist assistant reviews the medical record of a patient that sustained a brachial plexus injury. An entry by the patient's physician indicates that the posterior cord of the brachial plexus was severed. Which nerve would you expect to be the most seriously affected by the injury?

1. axillary
2. musculocutaneous
3. suprascapular
4. ulnar

118. A physical therapist assistant attempts to assess the strength of the tibialis posterior. To perform a manual muscle test, the therapist should position the lower extremity in:

1. eversion and dorsiflexion
2. inversion and dorsiflexion
3. eversion and plantar flexion
4. inversion and plantar flexion

119. A physical therapist assistant assesses a patient's posture using a plumb line. Assuming normal posture, which of the following would not be accurate in describing the relationship of the plumb line to a selected body part?

1. slightly anterior to the lateral malleolus
2. through the greater trochanter of the femur
3. posterior to the center of the knee
4. through the lobe of the ear

120. A physical therapist assistant performs a manual test of the triceps brachii. When performing the test, the therapist should offer resistance against the forearm in the direction of:

1. extension
2. flexion
3. supination
4. pronation

121. A physical therapist assistant works on bed mobility exercises with a patient recently diagnosed with cancer. The patient is extremely upset and tells her therapist, "I know I will never get better." The therapist's most appropriate response would be:

    1. Radiation treatments will make you feel much better.
    2. Many people have overcome larger obstacles.
    3. Having cancer must be very difficult for you to deal with.
    4. The exercises I show you can improve your condition.

122. There are a variety of different isolation categories which require the use of specific methods or techniques designed to reduce or prevent the transmission of disease or infection. Which of the following is required regardless of the specific isolation category?

    1. mask
    2. gown
    3. gloves
    4. hand washing

123. A patient is given a prescription for a nonsteroidal anti-inflammatory drug, which is to be administered three times a day with meals. What is the most common side effect of NSAIDs?

    1. convulsions
    2. fever
    3. nausea and vomiting
    4. stomach discomfort

124. A seven-month old infant demonstrates an abnormal persistence of the positive support reflex. Which therapeutic activity would not be limited by the presence of the reflex?

    1. crawl to stand transfer
    2. cruising
    3. plantigrade positioning using a bolster
    4. quadruped positioning and crawling

125. A patient with an IV in the antecubital region is treated in physical therapy. The physical therapist assistant would like to instruct the patient in upper extremity active range of motion exercises, but is concerned about placing excessive pressure on the infusion site. Which of the following exercises would not be indicated?

    1. shoulder abduction and adduction
    2. shoulder flexion and extension
    3. elbow flexion and extension
    4. wrist flexion and extension

126. A 42-year-old female that is unable to satisfactorily control the retention and release of urine uses a catheter. Which type of urinary catheter would not be appropriate for the patient?

    1. indwelling urinary catheter
    2. external urinary catheter
    3. Foley catheter
    4. suprapubic catheter

127. A physical therapist assistant performs an ultrasound treatment on a patient diagnosed with acute low back pain. When completing documentation using a S.O.A.P. note format, the therapist should record the treatment in the:

    1. subjective section
    2. objective section
    3. assessment section
    4. plan section

128. Accurate, clear, and concise documentation has become increasingly important for all health care providers. Which of the following suggestions to improve documentation would not be useful?

    1. avoid empty or open lines between entries in the medical record
    2. make sure all entries in the medical record are typewritten
    3. use abbreviations that have been standardized or accepted by a specific facility or the profession
    4. co-sign the entries of other medical personnel when necessary according to state and facility requirements

129. A patient, immediately after being transported outside the hospital to practice car transfers, informs the physical therapist assistant that he has to use the bathroom. The therapist's most appropriate response to meet the patient's physical need is to:

   1. ask the patient if it is an emergency
   2. complete the transfer training as quickly as possible and allow the patient to use the bathroom
   3. transport the patient back into the hospital to use the bathroom
   4. instruct the patient that in the future he should use the bathroom before beginning physical therapy

130. A physical therapist assistant examines a patient seven days status post total hip replacement. The patient's medical record indicates the surgeon utilized an anterolateral surgical approach. Which of the following motions would be the most important to restrict during the initial phase of rehabilitation?

   1. knee extension
   2. knee flexion
   3. hip lateral rotation
   4. hip medial rotation

131. A physical therapist assistant monitors a patient's pulse rate using the radial artery. Which of the following general statements regarding pulse rate is not accurate?

   1. pulse rate is increased with physical exertion
   2. pulse rate is decreased during relaxation or sleep
   3. pulse rate is decreased with anxiety or stress
   4. pulse rate is higher in children than adults

132. A patient informs a physical therapist assistant how frustrated she feels after being examined by her physician. The patient explains that she becomes so nervous, she cannot ask any questions during scheduled office visits. The therapist's most appropriate response is to:

   1. offer to go with the patient to her next scheduled physician visit
   2. offer to call the physician and ask any relevant questions
   3. suggest that the patient write down questions for the physician and bring them with her to the next scheduled visit
   4. tell the patient it is a very normal response to be nervous in the presence of a physician

133. An athlete is forced to contemplate knee surgery after spraining her anterior cruciate ligament playing soccer. Which situation would provide the most direct support for an anterior cruciate ligament reconstruction?

1. grade III ACL and grade I PCL injury
2. grade III ACL sprain with lateral meniscal involvement
3. grade II ACL sprain with medial meniscal involvement
4. functional instability

134. A patient with paraplegia is interested in learning how to perform a wheelie to assist with community mobility. The patient is independent with basic wheelchair propulsion. When instructing the patient to perform a wheelie, the physical therapist assistant should first teach the patient to:

1. make small adjustments (forward and backward) after being placed in the wheelie position
2. move into the wheelie position
3. perform turns while holding the wheelie position
4. statically hold the wheelie position after being placed in it by the therapist

135. A physical therapist assistant prepares a patient status post CVA with global aphasia for discharge from a rehabilitation hospital. The patient will be returning to her home with her husband and daughter. The most appropriate form of education to facilitate a safe discharge is to:

1. perform hands on training sessions with the patient and family
2. videotape the patient performing transfers and ADLs
3. provide written instructions on all ADLs and functional tasks
4. meet with family members to discuss the patient's present status and abilities

136. A physical therapist assistant assesses a patient's fine motor coordination following wrist surgery. Which of the following tasks would require the greatest amount of fine motor coordination?

1. stacking large blocks
2. assembling small bolts, nuts, and washers
3. turning cards
4. picking up large heavy objects

137. A physical therapist assistant monitors a patient's vital signs while exercising in a phase I cardiac rehabilitation program. The patient is status post myocardial infarction and has progressed without difficulty while involved in the program. Which of the following vital sign recordings would exceed the typical limits of a phase I program?

1. heart rate elevated 18 beats/minute above resting level
2. respiration rate = 25 breaths/minute
3. systolic blood pressure decreases by 20 mm Hg from resting level
4. diastolic blood pressure less than 100 mm Hg

138. A physical therapist assistant works with a patient that sustained an injury to the axillary nerve through the use of an assistive device. Which of the following ambulation aids would make the patient most susceptible to this type of injury?

1. walker
2. axillary crutches
3. Lofstrand crutches
4. parallel bars

139. A physical therapist assistant conducts a goniometric assessment of the wrist and hand. When determining the available range of motion for thumb flexion, the therapist should align the axis of the goniometer over the:

1. dorsal aspect of the first carpometacarpal joint
2. palmar aspect of the first carpometacarpal joint
3. midway between the dorsal aspect of the first and second carpometacarpal joints
4. midway between the palmar aspect of the first and second carpometacarpal joints

140. A physical therapist assistant works with a patient status post lower extremity amputation with a hip flexion contracture. Which amputation level would be most susceptible to a hip flexion contracture?

1. transfemoral
2. knee disarticulate
3. long transtibial knee
4. short transtibial knee

141. A physical therapist assistant treats a patient with post-polio syndrome. Given the patient's diagnosis, which of the following is the least likely impairment?

1. decreased strength
2. decreased sensation
3. decreased endurance
4. decreased functional mobility

142. A physical therapist assistant asks a patient who has been inconsistent with his attendance in physical therapy, why he is having difficulty keeping scheduled appointments. The patient responds that it is difficult to understand the scheduling card which lists the appointments. The therapist's most appropriate action would be to:

1. contact the referring physician to discuss the patient's poor attendance in therapy
2. make sure the patient is given a scheduling card at the conclusion of each session
3. write down the patient's appointments on a piece of paper in a manner which the patient can understand
4. discharge the patient since he is not interested in therapy

143. A variety of factors can influence blood pressure. Which individual would you expect to have the lowest systolic blood pressure?

1. 10-year-old male
2. 30-year-old female
3. 45-year-old female
4. 75-year-old male

144. An attorney contacts you by phone and requests specific information on a patient he claims to represent. Questions asked include the extent of the patient's disability and their willingness to return to work. The most appropriate response would be to:

1. answer the questions asked by the attorney
2. request the attorney to provide documented proof that he represents the patient and only then will you discuss the patient's situation
3. refer the attorney to the supervising physical therapist
4. instruct the attorney to complete the necessary paperwork and a copy of the patient's physical therapy records will be sent to the appropriate party

145. A physical therapist assistant employed in a rehabilitation hospital routinely works with an aide. Which of the following activities would not be appropriate for the aide to perform?

    1. cleaning and maintaining exercise equipment
    2. transporting patients
    3. preparing a treatment area
    4. developing an exercise program

146. A physical therapist assistant prepares to complete an assisted standing pivot transfer with a patient that requires moderate assistance. In order to increase a patient's independence with the transfer, which of the following instructions would be the most appropriate?

    1. I want you to help me perform the transfer.
    2. Try to utilize your own strength to complete the transfer.
    3. Only grab onto me if it is absolutely necessary.
    4. Use the power in your legs to assist you during the transfer.

147. A patient with spina bifida is referred to physical therapy for instruction in gait training. The patient exhibits good balance and coordination and has normal upper extremity strength. The patient uses a wheelchair as their primary mode of transportation and occasionally uses a swing-to gait pattern with Lofstrand crutches. The patient reports being frustrated by the lack of speed using the swing-to gait and would like to learn an alternate gait pattern. What gait pattern would be the most appropriate for the patient?

    1. two-point
    2. three-point
    3. swing-through
    4. four-point

148. A physical therapist assistant reviews the results of a lower extremity goniometric examination. Which of the following measurements would not be indicative of normal lower extremity range of motion?

    1. hip extension: 0 - 50 degrees
    2. knee flexion: 0 - 135 degrees
    3. ankle dorsiflexion: 0 - 20 degrees
    4. subtalar eversion: 0 - 5 degrees

149. A physical therapist assistant checks the water temperature in the hot pack unit after several patients report feeling excessive heat. Which temperature is most representative of the desired water temperature?

1. 135 degrees Fahrenheit
2. 150 degrees Fahrenheit
3. 160 degrees Fahrenheit
4. 180 degrees Fahrenheit

150. A physical therapist assistant utilizes a S.O.A.P. note format to complete daily documentation. Which of the following entries would not belong in the objective section?

1. describes onset of pain after lifting weight
2. ambulates with an assistive device independently
3. hot pack to thoracic spine for 20 minutes
4. right passive shoulder flexion range of motion is 128 degrees

Answer Key

1. Answer: 1   Resource: Kisner (p. 98)
The Valsalva maneuver is an attempt to forcibly exhale with the glottis, nose, and mouth closed. The action produces an increase in intrathoracic and intraabdominal pressures that leads to decreased venous blood flow to the heart. Patients most commonly utilize the Valsalva maneuver during heavy resistance exercise.

2. Answer: 4   Resource: O'Sullivan (p. 416)
Bridging occurs when a patient in hooklying lifts their buttocks and low back from a fixed surface. The activity can be used to facilitate pelvic motion and for strengthening of the hip extensors. Isometric gluteal sets are an appropriate precursor to bridging since the activity incorporates the hip extensors.

3. Answer: 2   Resource: Hillegass (p. 651)
Vibration is an airway clearance technique used in conjunction with postural drainage. The technique should be performed while the patient exhales following a deep inspiration. Vibration often causes the patient to produce a more effective cough.

4. Answer: 2   Resource: Hillegass (p. 433)
Incentive spirometry can assist patients to increase their maximal inspiration and prevent atelectasis. Normal values are 2,000-3,000 mL for females and 3,000-4,000 mL for males.

5. Answer: 2   Resource: Frownfelter (p. 755)
Incentive spirometry is designed to provide patients with visual or auditory feedback during deep inspiratory breathing. The device is used to prevent atelectasis in patients status post abdominal or thoracic surgery. Using the incentive spirometer once every two hours would be a fairly common schedule.

6. Answer: 1   Resource: Starkey (p. 293)
Spondylolisthesis refers to a condition where one vertebra slips forward on the one below it due to a bilateral fracture of the pars interarticularis. This condition most commonly occurs at L4-L5 or L5-S1. Children ages 10-15 who are involved in activities such as gymnastics, weightlifting, volleyball, and pole vaulting are particularly susceptible to spondylolisthesis.

7. Answer: 4   Resource: Brannon (p. 319)
Rating of perceived exertion provides a subjective measure of exercise intensity. Selected levels of perceived exertion using Borg's ten point scale: 0 - nothing, 3 - moderate, 5 - strong, 7 - very strong, 10 - very, very strong. Heart rate would not be an appropriate method to monitor exercise intensity due to the fixed rate pacemaker. Blood pressure and respiration rate are often monitored during exercise, however do not provide a measure of exercise intensity.

8. Answer: 3   Resource: O'Sullivan (p. 592)
The ankle-brachial index (ABI) is a ratio that is calculated by dividing the lower extremity pressure by the upper extremity pressure. Normal values of the ABI are 1.0 or slightly higher. Values less than .50 are indicative of severe arterial disease.

9. Answer: 2   Resource: Magee (p. 237)
A patient requires 30-70 degrees of horizontal adduction, 105-120 degrees of abduction, and 90 degrees of lateral rotation to independently comb his/her hair.

10. Answer: 3   Resource: Brunnstrom (p. 10)
Elbow flexion is usually the first and the strongest component of the flexor synergy.

11. Answer: 3   Resource: Goold (p. 32)
Positioning the patient in supine with the legs elevated would be inappropriate first aid management for a patient experiencing a CVA. This position may be warranted in a patient with hypovolemic shock.

12. Answer: 4   Resource: Pierson (p. 266)
Tiny air bubbles are a common occurrence in peripheral IV lines and are not necessarily indicative of any type of complication.

13. Answer: 3   Resource: Haggard (p. 83)
Lecture, handouts, and demonstration provide not only verbal and written information, but provide the target audience with the opportunity to observe an actual demonstration. This multitiered approach accomodates for a variety of learning styles.

14. Answer: 2   Resource: Norkin (p. 84)
Goniometric measurements of wrist flexion are conducted with the patient in sitting with the forearm supported on a firm surface.

15 Answer: 2   Resource: Magee (p. 801)
By maintaining the foot in a plantar flexed position the anterior talofibular ligament is positioned perpendicular to the long axis of the tibia. The talus should be moved anteriorly on the calcaneus after being placed in the test position.

16. Answer: 1   Resource: Magee (p. 801)
A positive anterior drawer test is indicative of a tear of the anterior talofibular ligament. When the talus is drawn forward there may be a dimple that appears over the area of the anterior talofibular ligament. Although the test is positive with isolated damage to the anterior talofibular ligament, anterior translation is greater when the damage is to both the anterior talofibular ligament and the calcaneofibular ligament.

17. Answer: 1   Resource: Magee (p. 364)
The boutonniere deformity is most frequently encountered in patients with rheumatoid arthritis or after trauma. It is caused by damage to the central tendinous slip of the extensor hood.

18. Answer: 3   Resource: Brannon (p. 106)
Patients with congestive heart failure may present with breathlessness, weakness, abdominal discomfort, and edema in the lower extremities resulting from venous stasis. Since sodium serves to retain water it is often restricted in a patient's diet.

19. Answer: 3   Resource: Kettenbach (p. 125)
Equipment needs and equipment ordered are typically included in the plan section of a S.O.A.P. note.

20. Answer: 3   Resource: Brannon (p. 316)
A perceived exertion scale is a subjective scale where patients rate the intensity of exercise.

21. Answer: 2   Resource: Goodman-Differential
                                                   Diagnosis (p. 25)
Open-ended questions guide the discussion, but do not restrict information to categories. Closed-ended questions are more impersonal and provide a limited number of response options.

22. Answer: 3   Resource: Ellis (p. 162)
All of the listed tasks are reasonable expectations for the patient, however moving from sitting to standing would be the most difficult due to the potential limitation in right knee range of motion as well as inadequate lower extremity strength.

23. Answer: 4   Resource: Pierson (p. 293)
Due to the probability associated with incidental contact, the front of the gown below waist level is considered to be non-sterile.

24. Answer: 3   Resource: Kendall (p. 208)
The medial hamstrings (semitendinosus, semimembranosus) muscles are tested with a patient in the prone position. The knee should be positioned between 50 and 70 degrees of flexion and the force should be applied in the direction of knee extension.

25. Answer: 3   Resource: Ellis (p. 15)
A supine position will ensure patient safety and allow the therapist full access to the residual limb.

26. Answer: 1   Resource: Pauls (p. 161)
Leaving the residual limb exposed to the air at all times would result in increased edema and a misshapened residual limb.

27. Answer: 4   Resource: Pierson (p. 267)
Positioning the collection bag on the cross brace beneath the seat will allow for it to be below the level of the bladder.

28 Answer: 2   Resource: Minor (p. 290)
The patient's balance and strength require the stability provided by a walker.

29. Answer: 4   Resource: O'Sullivan (p. 160)
Patients with cerebellar degeneration often exhibit hypotonia, not hypertonia.

30. Answer: 2   Resource: Davis (p. 119)
Inappropriate behavior is unacceptable and should not be tolerated, however the therapist needs to make the patient aware that her behavior is offensive.

31. Answer: 3   Resource: Davis (p. 88)
The response "surgery can be a very frightening thought" is an empathetic response that demonstrates respect for the patient's feelings.

32. Answer: 4   Resource: Brannon (p. 206)
Anxiety, tobacco, alcohol, and caffeine consumption can all serve to precipitate preventricular contractions. Sodium has not been shown to have any direct correlation with PVCs.

33. Answer: 2   Resource: Minor (p. 302)
Guarding should occur with one hand positioned on the patient's shoulder and the other on the hip. If a gait belt is used the lower hand should grasp the gait belt with the forearm in a supinated position.

34. Answer: 2   Resource: Levangie (p. 310)
The gluteus maximus and the hamstrings function as primary hip extensors. These muscles function in an eccentric fashion when moving from standing to sitting.

35. Answer: 2   Resource: Paz (p. 378)
Anemia refers to a reduction in the number of circulating red blood cells. Symptoms may include pallor, cyanosis, cool skin, vertigo, weakness, headache, and general malaise.

36. Answer: 2   Resource: Kisner (p. 550)
Patients that demonstrate an extension lag have greater passive extension than active extension. The difference in the passive and active extension range of motion is used to quantify the amount of the lag. Bony obstruction would not produce an extension lag since passive range of motion and active range of motion would be equal.

37. Answer: 4   Resource: Bickley (p. 228)
Wheezes are characterized by a high constant pitch during exhalation and are often indicative of narrowed airways or an airway obstruction. This condition is most commonly associated with asthma or bronchitis.

38. Answer: 2   Resource: Kendall (p. 221)
A manual muscle test of the gluteus medius should be performed with the patient in sidelying. The gluteus medius is a prime hip abductor.

39. Answer: 4   Resource: Standards of Practice
The physician is responsible for determining the patient's weight bearing status.

40. Answer: 4   Resource: Scott (p. 65)
Although a variety of subjective and objective data are admissible in a court of law, formal documentation is often paramount.

41. Answer: 3   Resource: Anderson (p. 469)
Effectiveness of the anterior drawer test is diminished by muscle guarding of the hamstrings which can obscure anterior displacement of the tibia. The anterior drawer test is performed with the patient in supine with 90 degrees of knee flexion. The Lachman test is performed with the patient in supine with 20-30 degrees of knee flexion.

42. Answer: 1   Resource: Minor (p. 368)
In order to allow the crutches to assist the involved leg the most appropriate sequence when descending stairs is crutches, involved leg, uninvolved leg.

43. Answer: 4   Resource: Umphred (p. 494)
Patients with an injury at the L1 level typically have normal proprioception at the hip and limited spasticity. Patients can become functional ambulators using knee-ankle-foot orthoses and forearm crutches.

44. Answer: 2   Resource: Saunders (p. 276)
Studies have demonstrated that disc protrusion can be reduced and spinal nerve root compression symptoms relieved through the use of spinal traction.

45. Answer: 2   Resource: Robinson (p. 160)
When stimulated over a motor point a normally innervated muscle will exhibit a brisk contraction followed by a rapid relaxation. The motor point of a muscle generally refers to the location on the muscle belly where the motor nerve enters.

46. Answer: 1   Resource: Pierson (p. 109)
Sitting in a low chair may increase hip flexion beyond the established parameters for patients following hip replacement surgery.

47. Answer: 4   Resource: Michlovitz (p. 81)
Systemic vasoconstrictors cause smooth muscle contraction and decreased vessel diameter resulting in diminished blood flow.

48. Answer: 1   Resource: Buchanan (p. 227)
Heterotopic ossification refers to abnormal bone growth in tissue. Signs and symptoms include decreased range of motion, local swelling, and warmth. Heterotopic ossification often occurs in patients following a head injury.

49. Answer: 1   Resource: Shamus (p. 400)
The injury mechanism associated with an acromioclavicular injury is a direct blow to the tip of the shoulder which serves to displace the acromion inferior to the clavicle.

50. Answer: 3   Resource: Guide to Physical Therapist
                                                    Practice (S31)
Physical therapist assistants perform procedures and related tasks that have been selected and delegated by the supervising physical therapist. It is not appropriate to delegate an examination.

51. Answer: 4   Resource: Michlovitz (p. 142)
A warm water bath can be a source of superficial heat and is readily accessible in all homes.

52. Answer: 3   Resource: Norkin (p. 222)
The active range of motion available in the right knee (20 - 70 degrees) is extremely limited. Average knee flexion according to the American Academy of Orthopedic Surgeons is 0 - 135 degrees.

53. Answer: 2   Resource: Rothstein (p. 24)
An entrance ramp that is six inches in length for each inch of vertical rise is too steep. A properly constructed ramp should be a minimum of 12 inches in length for each inch of rise.

54. Answer: 2   Resource: Norkin (p. 41)
Intrarater reliability refers to the amount of agreement between repeated measures of the same joint position by an individual therapist.

55. Answer: 1   Resource: Magee (p. 691)
The iliotibial band serves as a secondary restraint to the anterior cruciate ligament.

56. Answer: 3   Resource: O'Sullivan (p. 802)
A patient's question should be answered in a direct and forthcoming manner whenever possible. Frequent repetition is a component of any treatment plan for patients with short-term memory loss.

57. Answer: 1   Resource: Hertfelder (p. 138)
Recommendations when seated at a computer terminal include: thighs positioned parallel with the floor, top of the screen at eye level, minimum viewing distance 12 inches, height of the work surface 23-28 inches, and width of the work surface 30 inches.

58. Answer: 4   Resource: Robinson (p. 182)
A Milwaukee brace is a common orthotic device used to treat children with progressive scoliosis. The brace is designed to improve alignment in the developing spine and is usually worn until spinal growth ceases.

59. Answer: 1   Resource: Magee (p. 811)
Anterior compartment syndrome often affects the deep peroneal nerve as it passes under the extensor retinaculum. The result of nerve compression ranges from a mild sensory disturbance to an inability to dorsiflex the foot.

60. Answer: 4   Resource: Arnheim (p. 107)
The triceps and the subscapular skinfolds are the two most common sites utilized when measuring body composition using a skinfold caliper. Other possible sites include the iliac crest, anterior chest, just below and lateral to the umbilicus, and the anterior thigh.

61. Answer: 2   Resource: Magee (p. 187)
Restricted mouth opening would be characteristic of an anterior disk dislocation that does not reduce. A loud click or pop would be consistent with an anterior disk dislocation that does reduce.

62. Answer: 3   Resource: Kisner (p. 301)
Active stretching exercises are contraindicated since the patient is in the acute inflammatory phase. Limited motion in a joint during this phase may be due to fluid in the joint space and not adhesions. Stretching may serve to exacerbate the patient's condition and perhaps result in hypermobility. Although therapists rarely view immobilization as a component of a patient care plan, in this particular instance it may be advisable.

63. Answer: 2   Resource: Kendall (p. 193)
    The flexor digitorum brevis acts to flex the proximal interphalangeal joints and
    assists in flexion of the metatarsophalangeal joints of the second through fifth
    digits.

64. Answer: 1   Resource: Umphred (p. 492)
    Self range of motion of the lower extremities is a realistic goal at the C7 level, but
    not at the C5 level.

65. Answer: 4   Resource: Guide for Conduct of the
                                                         Physical Therapist Assistant
    Therapists should never place their personal safety in jeopardy.

66. Answer: 4   Resource: Goodman-Differential
                                                         Diagnosis (p. 38)
    An open-ended question allows for a myriad of responses. The question "How
    well are you able to complete assigned activities?" provides the patient with the
    opportunity to provide specific information. The other remaining options are
    examples of closed-ended questions.

67. Answer: 1   Resource: Norkin (p. 63)
    When measuring lateral shoulder rotation the axis of the goniometer is placed
    over the olecranon process. The stationary arm is perpendicular to the floor and
    the moving arm is aligned with the ulna using the olecranon and ulnar styloid for
    reference.

68. Answer: 4   Resource: Kendall (p. 277)
    The upper fibers of the pectoralis major are innervated by the lateral pectoral
    nerve C5, C6, C7.

69. Answer: 4   Resource: Pierson (p. 148)
    The elbow is not typically in direct contact with a given component of a
    wheelchair and is therefore not likely to be the site of a pressure ulcer.

70. Answer: 1   Resource: Magee (p. 529)
    Segmental levels for deep tendon reflexes: Achilles S1-S2, lateral hamstrings S1-
    S2, patellar L3-L4, posterior tibial L4-L5.

71. Answer: 3   Resource: O'Sullivan (p. 800)
    Patients in the confused-agitated stage have a short attention span and therefore
    require numerous activities to be included in each treatment session.

72. Answer: 4   Resource: Paz (p. 630)
    Vocational dysfunction is not associated with pressure sores. Other risk factors
    include nutritional deficiencies, incontinence, depression, diminished sensation,
    infection, spasticity, and disuse atrophy.

73. Answer: 4   Resource: O'Sullivan (p. 861)
Splinting in elbow extension and forearm supination will effectively limit contractures and maximize functional use of the upper extremity.

74. Answer: 2   Resource: Hoppenfeld (p. 122)
C7 level: Motor - triceps, wrist flexors, finger extensors
            Sensation - middle finger
            Reflex - triceps

75. Answer: 3   Resource: Umphred (p. 804)
Changing the patient's environment and staff frequently will yield greater levels of stress and cognitive dysfunction.

76. Answer: 3   Resource: Pauls (p. 654)
Osteoporosis refers to a disease process that results in a reduction of bone mass. Screening by measuring height can provide an inexpensive method to screen for this disease.

77. Answer: 3   Resource: O'Sullivan (p. 669)
A patient walking at a comfortable pace with a transfemoral prosthesis requires nearly 50% more oxygen than normal. This value is significantly higher than the other stated options.

78. Answer: 1   Resource: Standards of Practice
The highest priority should be to direct attention toward the unattended patient exercising in the gym. It is essential to make sure the patient is not a safety risk.

79. Answer: 3   Resource: Garrison (p. 120)
Patients who have sustained a cardiac event often exercise at an intensity of 60% of the maximal heart rate obtained on a symptom-limited exercise treadmill test.

80. Answer: 2   Resource: Kisner (p. 97)
Reducing the weight to ten pounds will allow the patient to maintain the integrity of the originally prescribed exercise while allowing the patient to perform the exercise correctly.

81. Answer: 4   Resource: Kisner (p. 714)
Patients with chronic arterial insufficiency typically have diminished blood flow and resultant ischemia. Positioning with the legs elevated will only serve to exacerbate the patient's symptoms.

82. Answer: 4   Resource: Pauls (p. 329)
Guillain-Barre is an acute polyneuropathy causing rapid, progressive loss of motor function. Although mild sensory loss can be evident, absent sensation is extremely rare.

83. Answer: 1   Resource: Kettenbach (p. 125)
The word "will" denotes future tense. This entry is most appropriate in the plan
section of a S.O.A.P. note.

84. Answer: 3   Resource: Goodman – Pathology
                                                                    (p. 455)
A progressive ambulation program can be extremely beneficial for patients with
peripheral arterial disease. During the initial stages of the program the therapist
should instruct the patient to rest when they experience signs and symptoms of
claudication. As the patient becomes more familiar with the program the therapist
may elect to have the patient continue walking through tolerable levels of pain.

85. Answer: 1   Resource: Goodman – Pathology
                                                                    (p. 307)
Positioning the patient in supine with the knees extended and the toes pointing
toward the ceiling maintains the hips, knees, and ankles in an optimal position and
therefore reduces the likelihood of a lower extremity contracture.

86. Answer: 1   Resource: Minor (p. 294)
A rolling walker provides the patient with the necessary stability to ambulate
safely. The wheels allow for a smoother more coordinated gait pattern.

87. Answer: 2   Resource: Magee (p. 632)
This scenario describes Ely's test which if positive is indicative of tightness of the
two joint hip flexor (rectus femoris).

88. Answer: 2   Resource: Magee (p. 621)
Anteversion refers to the degree of angulation of the neck of the femur. In adults
the mean is 8-15 degrees. Patients with excessive anteversion often exhibit more
than 60 degrees of hip medial rotation and decreased lateral rotation.

89. Answer: 3   Resource: Norkin (p. 36)
Reliability refers to the amount of consistency between successive measurements.
Since the question indicates a single therapist performing successive
measurements, the form of reliability should be termed intrarater.

90. Answer: 4   Resource: Gross (p. 127)
The bowel is associated with the sacral segments of the spinal cord S2-S4. The
Achilles reflex is from the S1 level. Sensation in the area of the posterior calf is
from the S1-S2 level.

91. Answer: 2   Resource: O'Sullivan (p. 268)
The hip is required to flex during initial swing to allow for proper clearance and
advancement of the limb during gait. Normally, dorsiflexion also occurs.
Without the use of the dorsiflexors the hip flexors need to be strengthened in
order to attain proper clearance.

92. Answer: 2   Resource: Sullivan (p. 71)
Bridging causes the muscles of the low back and hip extensors to isometrically contract. The activity is often required for independent bed mobility and serves to promote hip stability.

93. Answer: 3   Resource: Magee (p. 631)
Patients with tight hip flexors often exhibit an increased lordosis. Shortness of the hip flexors is observed in standing as lumbar lordosis with an anterior pelvic tilt or it can be assessed using the Thomas test.

94. Answer: 3   Resource: Magee (p. 629)
Measuring from the medial knee joint line to the medial malleolus allows for an independent assessment of tibial length and also avoids any potential asymmetries due to leg girth.

95. Answer: 2   Resource: Magee (p. 225)
Normal shoulder complex abduction = 180 degrees. Approximately 120 degrees of movement occurs at the glenohumeral joint and 60 degrees at the scapulothoracic articulation. The question specifically asks about glenohumeral abduction.

96. Answer: 2   Resource: Ratliffe (p. 47)
The activities the child can perform occur between three and four years of age in normal development. The activities the child cannot perform typically occur between five and seven years of age.

97. Answer: 4   Resource: Minor (p. 54)
Once a nonsterile object is placed within a sterile field, the entire sterile field should be considered nonsterile.

98. Answer: 3   Resource: Norkin (p. 26)
An entry in the medical record needs to be as clear and concise as possible. The question indicates that the patient can flex his right shoulder to 178 degrees, however does not identify if the patient was able to achieve a starting position of 0. It is always necessary to state the direction of the movement and whether it was active or passive motion.

99. Answer: 3   Resource: Rothstein (p. 995)
Protective asepsis for respiratory isolation includes a mask. Examples of conditions that may require respiratory isolation include measles, mumps, and pertussis.

100. Answer: 4   Resource: Ratliffe (p. 29)
Assuming a sitting position independently occurs at 6 - 7 months of age.
Creeping on hands and knees and cruising along furniture occur at 8 - 9 months.
Pulling to standing from a half kneel position occurs at 10 - 11 months.

101. Answer: 2   Resource: Bickley (p. 600)
Wernicke's aphasia refers to an inability to comprehend written or spoken words.
As a result of this condition it is inappropriate to provide detailed instructions.

102. Answer: 1   Resource: Minor (p. 288)
The parallel bars provide the most stable setting for the patient to begin
ambulation activities.

103. Answer: 4   Resource: Pierson (p. 194)
A walker with a platform attachment will provide the stability the patient requires
while avoiding significant pressure on both of the fracture sites.

104. Answer: 2   Resource: Pierson (p. 123)
A sliding board transfer is possible based on the patient's upper extremity
strength. The transfer will allow the patient to maintain a high level of
independence.

105. Answer: 3   Resource: Hoppenfeld (p. 101)
The flexor digitorum profundus is responsible for flexing the distal
interphalangeal joint of the four fingers and assisting with flexion of the proximal
interphalangeal and metacarpophalangeal joints.

106. Answer: 2   Resource: Bly (p. 63)
Rolling from prone to supine usually occurs in the fifth month, while rolling from
supine to prone occurs in the sixth month.

107. Answer: 3   Resource: Rothstein (p. 44)
The minimum knee clearance required for a wheelchair to be positioned under a
sink is 29 inches.

108. Answer: 2   Resource: O'Sullivan (p. 899)
A patient with T10 paraplegia would utilize a wheelchair for functional mobility
due to the lack of active motion in the lower extremities and the high energy cost
of ambulation with bracing and an assistive device.

109. Answer: 4   Resource: Norkin (p. 72)
The therapist should stabilize the distal end of the humerus in order to prevent
shoulder flexion.

110. Answer: 2   Resource: O'Sullivan (p. 632)

Positioning in supine with the residual limb elevated on a pillow will reinforce hip flexion and may lead to a contracture. Periodic prone positioning is useful to avoid the development of a hip flexion contracture.

111. Answer: 2   Resource: Minor (p. 299)

A three-point gait pattern is used by patients who have one involved lower extremity. The gait pattern most commonly is performed with two crutches or a walker.

112. Answer: 2   Resource: Minor (p. 296)

Although axillary crutches do not offer the stability offered by parallel bars or a walker, they provide good stability and support.

113. Answer: 4   Resource: Michlovitz (p. 157)

Water temperature for patients with cardiovascular or pulmonary disease should not exceed 38 degrees Celsius. Thirty seven degrees Celsius is equivalent to normal body temperature.

114. Answer: 4   Resource: Michlovitz (p. 101)

Studies have not identified any adverse effects from the use of cryotherapy over epiphyseal areas in children.

115. Answer: 4   Resource: Magee (p. 410)

The location of the radial pulse can also be described as being situated between the tendons of the flexor carpi radialis and abductor pollicis longus.

116. Answer: 4   Resource: Haggard (p. 112)

Since the therapist is providing specific instructions regarding the frequency and duration of each exercise, it is essential to provide written instructions. Demonstrating an exercise to a patient can promote increased understanding and compliance.

117. Answer: 1   Resource: Rothstein (p. 303)

The axillary nerve descends from the posterior cord of the brachial plexus. The axillary nerve innervates the deltoid and teres minor muscles.

118. Answer: 4   Resource: Kendall (p. 202)

The lower leg should be positioned in plantar flexion and inversion. Resistance should be applied against the medial side and plantar surface of the foot in the direction of dorsiflexion of the ankle joint and eversion of the foot. The tibialis posterior is innervated by the tibial nerve.

119. Answer: 3   Resource: Kendall (p. 75)

A plumb line should fall slightly anterior to a midline through the knee in a patient with ideal alignment.

120. Answer: 2   Resource: Kendall (p. 270)
The triceps brachii serves to extend the forearm, therefore resistance should be applied against the forearm in the direction of flexion. The triceps brachii is innervated by the radial nerve.

121. Answer: 3   Resource: Davis (p. 88)
The statement "having cancer must be very difficult for you to deal with" shows compassion for the patient's current condition without offering a false sense of hope. It may also serve to provide a platform for the patient to express their feelings.

122. Answer: 4   Resource: Pierson (p. 276)
Hand washing should be performed before and after providing patient care. This relatively simple task can offer protection against the spread of infection for patients and health care professionals.

123. Answer: 4   Resource: Ciccone (p. 201)
Gastrointestinal distress is the most common side effect of NSAIDs. There are a large variety of medications which are labeled as NSAIDs. Some such as aspirin have been shown to yield more gastrointestinal irritation than some of the more recent NSAIDs.

124. Answer: 4   Resource: Ratliffe (p. 27)
The positive support reflex is elicited through weight bearing on the balls of the feet while standing.

125. Answer: 3   Resource: Pierson (p. 266)
The antecubital area refers to the cubital fossa on the volar surface of the elbow. Elbow flexion and extension would result in significant pressure on the infusion site.

126. Answer: 2   Resource: Pierson (p. 268)
External catheters are applied over the shaft of a penis and are therefore inappropriate for females.

127. Answer: 2   Resource: Kettenbach (p. 44)
Treatment performed during a physical therapy session should be documented in the objective section of a S.O.A.P. note.

128. Answer: 2   Resource: Kettenbach (p. 8)
Although typewritten entries in the medical record are acceptable, they are not required.

129. Answer: 3   Resource: Standards of Ethical Conduct
                                                        for the Physical Therapist
                                                        Assistant
The only viable solution to meet the patient's physical need is to allow him to use the bathroom.

130. Answer: 3   Resource: Pierson (p. 109)
A patient status post total hip replacement using an anterolateral surgical approach would be most restricted in lateral rotation. Failure to restrict lateral rotation may result in hip dislocation or subluxation. A posterolateral surgical approach would restrict medial rotation.

131. Answer: 3   Resource: Pierson (p. 50)
Pulse rate is increased with anxiety or stress.

132. Answer: 3   Resource: Davis (p. 85)
Suggesting the patient write down questions for the physician is a practical and realistic option that will assist her in future interactions.

133. Answer: 4   Resource: Kisner (p. 535)
Many individuals are able to continue to function at high levels despite a variety of ligamentous and meniscal injuries, therefore functional instability provides the most direct support for an anterior cruciate ligament reconstruction.

134. Answer: 4   Resource: Buchanan (p. 139)
Statically holding the wheelie position after being placed in it by the therapist requires the least skill and will provide the patient with the opportunity to gain a sense of balance before moving to more difficult activities.

135. Answer: 1   Resource: Haggard (p. 74)
Hands on training sessions provide unique opportunities for the therapist to assess the competence of family members in a structured environment.

136. Answer: 2   Resource: Magee (p. 386)
Assembling small bolts, nuts, and washers are activities used in a number of assessment measures which examine fine motor coordination such as the Purdue Peg Board Test.

137. Answer: 3   Resource: Brannon (p. 3)
Systolic blood pressure typically increases during exercise, therefore a reduction of 20 mm Hg from an established resting value would be unacceptable.

138. Answer: 2   Resource: Minor (p. 340)
Patients using axillary crutches often lean forward on the crutches to support the body during periods of standing. This activity can lead to damage in the axillary region.

139. Answer: 2   Resource: Norkin (p. 104)
Carpometacarpal flexion occurs in a frontal plane around an anterior-posterior axis with the patient in the anatomical position.

140. Answer: 1   Resource: Ellis (p. 12)
Frequent prone positioning is important for patients with transfemoral and transtibial amputations, however patients with transfemoral amputations are more susceptible to a hip flexion contracture.

141. Answer: 2   Resource: Paz (p. 334)
Post-polio syndrome is a term used to describe symptoms that occur years after the onset of poliomyelitis. The condition is believed to result as remaining motor units become more dysfunctional. Sensation is not typically affected by post-polio syndrome.

142. Answer: 3   Resource: Davis (p. 85)
In order to determine if the patient's poor attendance in therapy is due to difficulty understanding the scheduling card, the information must be presented in a manner that the patient can understand.

143. Answer: 1   Resource: Rothstein (p. 592)
Blood pressure tends to increase with age. Average blood pressure for a 10-year-old male is 90/60 mm Hg.

144. Answer: 3   Resource: Standards of Practice
The supervising physical therapist should speak to the attorney. Patient information should not be released until the attorney has completed the necessary paperwork and the patient has signed a release of medical information form.

145. Answer: 4   Resource: Guide to Physical Therapist
                                                    Practice (p. S32)
The physical therapy aide is a non-licensed worker who is trained under the direction of a physical therapist. Aides are involved in patient related and non-patient related duties as delegated by physical therapists and physical therapist assistants, however would not be responsible for developing an exercise program.

146. Answer: 2   Resource: Davis (p. 87)
"Try to utilize your own strength to complete the transfer" is a direct statement which should present the patient with a clear understanding of the therapist's objective. It also places the patient in an active instead of a passive position.

147. Answer: 3   Resource: Minor (p. 299)
A swing-through gait pattern relies on the same principles as a swing-to gait pattern, however allows a patient to bring the lower extremities beyond the point to which the assistive devices were advanced.

148. Answer: 1   Resource: Norkin (p. 222)
    According to the Academy of Orthopedic Surgeons normal hip extension is 0-30 degrees.

149. Answer: 3   Resource: Michlovitz (p. 116)
    Hot packs are stored in units that have a water temperature of approximately 160 degrees Fahrenheit or 71.1 degrees Celsius.

150. Answer: 1   Resource: Kettenbach (p. 45)
    The objective section of a S.O.A.P. note is typically reserved for the results of measurements and objective observations. The entry "describes onset of pain after lifting weight" would belong in the subjective section.

Appendix

Performance Analysis Summary

	Available Questions	Correct Questions	% Correct
Time Management Exercise	50		
Content Outline Exercise	80		
Sample Examination Exercise	150		
Total	280		

Time Management Diagnostic Sheet

	Day One	Day Two	Day Three	Total
CLASS				
STUDY				
INDIVIDUAL TIME				
SOCIAL TIME				
EXERCISE				
WORK				
SLEEP				
NAP				
SPECIAL APPOINTMENT				

Activity Log

	Day One	Day Two	Day Three
8:00			
9:00			
10:00			
11:00			
12:00			
1:00			
2:00			
3:00			
4:00			
5:00			
6:00			
7:00			
8:00			
9:00			

Relaxation Exercise

Periodically as indicated by your learning style, use the sample relaxation exercise to relieve your body of unwanted anxiety and stress. Each of the steps should be completed in a slow and somewhat exaggerated manner.

1. Take a deep breath and expire slowly.

2. Close your eyes tightly for 10 seconds and slowly open them.

3. Lift your shoulders towards your ears.

4. Make a tight fist and flex your elbows.

5. Squeeze your buttocks tightly and hold for 3 seconds.

6. Extend your knees and plantar flex your ankles.

7. Close your eyes tightly for 10 seconds and slowly open them.

8. Take a deep breath and expire slowly.

Resource List

American Physical Therapy Association
1111 North Fairfax Street
Alexandria, Virginia 22314
Phone: (800) 999-2782
Web site: www.apta.org
Fax on demand: (800) 399-2782

Federation of State Boards of Physical Therapy
509 Wythe Street
Alexandria, Virginia 22314
Phone: (703) 299-3100
Web site: www.fsbpt.org

Mainely Physical Therapy
P.O. Box 7242
Scarborough, Maine 04070-7242
Toll Free: (866) PTEXAMS
Phone: (207) 885-0304
Web site: www.ptexams.com
Fax: (207) 883-8377

Physical Therapy State Licensing Agencies

Alabama

Alabama Board of Physical Therapy
100 N. Union Street
Suite 627
Montgomery, AL 36130-5040

(334) 242-4064
www.pt.state.al.us

Arizona

Arizona State Board of Physical Therapy
1400 West Washington
Suite 230
Phoenix, AZ 85007

(602) 542-3095
www.ptboard.state.az.us

California

PT Board of California
1418 Howe Avenue
Suite 16
Sacramento, CA 95825

(916) 561-8200
www.ptb.ca.gov

Connecticut

Connecticut Dept of Public Health
410 Capitol Avenue
MS #12APP
Hartford, CT 06134-0308

(860) 509-7590
www.state.ct.us/dph/

Alaska

State PT & OT Board Div of Occup Licensing
333 Willoughby Avenue, 9th Floor
P.O. Box 110806
Juneau, AK 99811

(907) 465-2580
www.dced.state.ak.us/occ/pphy.htm

Arkansas

Arkansas State Board of Physical Therapy
9 Shackleford Plaza
Suite 3
Little Rock, AR 72211

(501) 228-7100
www.arptb.org

Colorado

Colorado Division of Registrations
1560 Broadway
Suite 1545
Denver, CO 80202

(303) 894-2440
www.dora.state.co.us/Physical-Therapy

Delaware

Division of Professional Regulation
861 Silver Lake Blvd.
Suite 203 Cannon Building
Dover, DE 19904-2467

(302) 744-4506
www.state.de.us/research/profreg/physical.htm

District of Columbia

DC Board of Physical Therapy
Dept of Health
825 N. Capital Street, NE, Rm 2224
Washington, DC 20002

(202) 442-4764

Georgia

Georgia Board of Physical Therapy
237 Coliseum Drive
Macon, GA 31217

(912) 207-1620
www.sos.state.ga.us/plb/pt/

Idaho

ID State Board of Medicine
1755 Westgate Drive
Suite 140
Boise, ID 83704

(208) 327-7000
www.bom.state.id.us

Indiana

Indiana Physical Therapy Committee
402 W. Washington Street
Room W041
Indianapolis, IN 46204

(317) 234-2051
www.in.gov/hpb/boards/ptc/

Florida

Dept of Health, MQA, Board of Physical Therapy
Practice
4052 Bald Cypress Way
Bin #C05
Tallahassee, FL 32399-3255

(850) 245-4373
www.doh.state.fl.us/mqa

Hawaii

Dept of Commerce & Consumer Affairs
P.O. Box 3469
Honolulu, HI 96801

(808) 586-2694

Illinois

Dept of Professional Regulation
320 West Washington
3rd Floor
Springfield, IL 62786

(217) 782-8556
www.dpr.state.il.us

Iowa

Board of Physical & Occupational Therapy
Examiners
Iowa Dept of Public Health
321 East 12th Street, 5th Floor
Des Moines, IA 50319-0075

(515) 281-4413

Kansas

KS State Board of Healing Arts
PT Examining Committee
235 S. Topeka Blvd
Topeka, KS 66603

(785) 296-7413
www.ink.org/public/boha

Louisiana

LA State Board of PT Examiners
714 E. Kaliste Saloom Road
Suite D2
Lafayette, LA 70508-3834

(337) 262-1043
www.laptboard.org

Maryland

Board of Physical Therapy Examiners
4201 Patterson Avenue #318
Baltimore, MD 21215-2299

(410) 764-4752
www.dhmh.state.md.us/bphte/

Michigan

Physical Therapy State Boards
P.O. Box 30670
Lansing, MI 48909

(517) 335-0918
www.cis.state.mi.us/bhser/home.htm

Mississippi

MS State Dept of Health Div of Licensure & Reg
Professional Licensure Rm 160
570 East Woodrow Wilson Blvd
Jackson, MS 39216

(601) 576-7262

Kentucky

Kentucky State Board of PT
9110 Leesgate Road, #6
Louisville, KY 40222-5159

(502) 327-8497
www.kbpt.state.ky.us

Maine

Board of Examiners in PT
35 State House Station
Augusta, ME 04330

(207) 624-8600
www.state.me.us/pfr/led/ledhome2.htm

Massachusetts

MA Board of Allied Health Professionals
Division of Registration
239 Causeway Street, Suite 500
Boston, MA 02114

(617) 727-3071
www.state.ma.us/reg/boards/ah

Minnesota

MN Board of Physical Therapy
2829 University Avenue, SE, #315
Minneapolis, MN 55414-3222

(612) 627-5406
www.physicaltherapy.state.mn.us

Missouri

Advisory Comm for Prof PTs & PTAs
P.O. Box 4
3605 Missouri Boulevard
Jefferson City, MO 65102

(573) 751-0098
www.ded.state.mo.us

Montana

Board of Physical Therapy Examiners
301 South Park, 4th Floor
P.O. Box 200513
Helena, MT 59620-0513

(406) 841-2369

Nevada

NV State Bd of Physical Therapy Examiners
3150 W. Sahara Ane.
Suite B-13
Las Vegas, NV 89102

(702) 876-5535

New Jersey

NJ State Board of PT
P.O. Box 45014
Newark, NJ 07101

(937) 504-6455

New York

State Board for PT
89 Washington Avenue
Education Bldg, East Mezzanine
Albany, NY 12234

(518) 474-3817
www.op.nysed.gov/pt.htm

Nebraska

Board of Physical Therapy
301 Centennial Mall
P.O. Box 94986
Lincoln, NE 68509

(402) 471-0547
www.hhs.state.ne.us/lis/lis.asp

New Hampshire

PT Governing Boad of NH
Office of Allied Health Prof
2 Industrial Park Drive
Concord, NH 03301

(603) 271-8389

New Mexico

NM Physical Therapy Board
2055 S. Pacheco
Suite 400
Santa Fe, NM 87505

(505) 476-7085
www.state.nm.us/rid/b&c/ptb

North Carolina

North Carolina Board of Physical Therapy
18 W. Colony Place #140
Durham, NC 27705

(919) 490-6393
www.ncptboard

North Dakota

ND State Examination Committee for PT
106 Eastern Avenue
Grafton, ND 58237

(701) 352-1621

Oklahoma

Bd of Med Lic & Sup
PT Advisory Committee
5104 North Francis, Suite C
Oklahoma City, OK 73118

(405) 848-6841
www.osbmls.state.ok.us

Pennsylvania

PA State Board of PT
P.O. Box 2649
Harrisburg, PA 17105

(717) 783-7134
www.dos.state.pa.us

Rhode Island

Rhode Island PT Board
Division of Prof Regulation
3 Capitol Hill, Room 104
Providence, RI 02908-5097

(401) 222-2827
www.health.state.ri.us

South Dakota

SD Board of Medical Examiners
1323 S. Minnesota Avenue
Sioux Falls, SD 57105

(605) 334-8343

Ohio

Ohio State Board of Physical and Occupational
Therapy
77 S. High Street
16th Floor
Columbus, OH 43215-6108

(614) 466-3774
www.state.oh.us/pyt

Oregon

PT Licensing Board
800 NE Oregon Street
Suite 407
Portland, OR 97232

(503) 731-4047
www.ptboard.state.or.us

Puerto Rico

Office of Regulation and Certification
Call Box 10200
Santurce, PR 00908

(787) 725-8161 x209

South Carolina

Board of PT Examiners
110 Centerview Drive
P.O. Box 11329
Columbia, SC 29211

(803) 896-4655
www.llr.state.sc.us

Tennessee

Div of Health Related Boards
Bd of Occupational & Physical Therapy
426 5th Ave North, 1st Floor
Nashville, TN 37247

(615) 532-5136
www.state.tn.us/health/links.html

Texas

TX Board of PT Examiners
1308 Queenspark
Austin, TX 78701

(903) 531-4330
www.ecptote.state.tx.us

Vermont

Physical Therapy Advisors
Office of Professional Regulations
26 Terrace Street, Drawer 09
Montpelier, VT 05609-1106

(802) 828-2390
www.sec.state.vt.us

Virginia

Board of Physical Therapy
Dept of Health Professions, 5th Floor
6603 West Broad Street
Richmond , VA 23230

(804) 662-9924

West Virginia

WV Board of Physical Therapy
153 W. Main Street
Suite 103
Clarksburg, WV 26301

(304) 627-2251

Wyoming

WY Board of Physical Therapy
2020 Carey Avenue
Suite 201
Cheyenne, WY 82002

(307) 777-3507

Utah

Division of Professional Licensing
160 East 300 South
Salt Lake City, UT 84114

(801) 530-6632

Virgin Islands

VI Board of PT Examiners
48 Sugar Estate
St. Thomas, VI 00802

(340) 774-0117

Washington

Washington Bd of PT
1112 SE Quince Street
P.O. Box 47868
Olympia, WA 98504-7868

(360) 236-4700
www.doh.wa.gov/hsqa/hpqad/physical_ther

Wisconsin

WI Dept of Regulation & Licensing
Rm 178, 1400 E. Washington Avenue
P.O. Box 8935
Madison, WI 53708-8935

(608) 266-2112

Prometric Testing Centers

Alaska
Anchorage

Alabama
Birmingham
Decatur
Dothan
Mobile
Montgomery

Arkansas
Arkadelphia
Fort Smith
Little Rock

Arizona
Goodyear
Phoenix
Tucson

California
Anaheim
Atascadero
Brea\Fullerton
Culver City (3)
Diamond Bar
Fair Oaks
Fremont
Gardena
Glendale (2)
Irvine
La Mesa
Palm Desert
Piedmont
Rancho Cucamonga
Redlands
Riverside
San Diego
San Francisco (2)
San Jose (2)
Santa Rosa
Walnut Creek
Westlake Village

Colorado
Boulder
Colorado Springs
Denver
Glendale
Pueblo

Connecticut
Glastonbury
Hamden
Norwalk

District of Columbia
Washington, D.C.

Delaware
Dover
Wilmington

Florida
Cassellberry
Fort Myers
Gainesville
Hollywood
Jacksonville
Maitland
Miami Lakes
Sarasota (2)
Tallahassee
Tampa
Temple Terrace

Georgia
Albany
Atlanta (2)
Augusta
Jonesboro
Macon
Savannah
Marietta (2)
Valdosta

Hawaii
Honolulu (temp)
Kailua

Iowa
Ames
Bettendorf
Sioux City
West Des Moines

Idaho
Boise

Illinois
Carbondale
Chicago (3)
Homewood
Lombard
Northbrook
Peoria
Springfield
Sycamore
Westchester

Indiana
Evansville
Fort Wayne
Indianapolis (2)
Lafayette
Merrillville
Mishawaka
Terre Haute

Kansas
Topeka
Wichita

Kentucky
Lexington
Louisville

Louisiana
Baton Rouge
Bossier City
New Orleans

Massachusetts
Boston (2)
Braintree
Brookline
East Longmeadow
Lexington
Waltham (2)
Worcester (2)

Maryland
Baltimore
Bethesda
Columbia
Lanham
Pikesville
Salisbury

Maine
Orono
South Portland

Michigan
Detroit\Southfield
Grand Rapids
Lansing
Livonia
Portage
Troy
Utica

Minnesota
Bloomington (3)
Duluth
Rochester
St. Cloud
Woodbury

Missouri
Ballwin
Cape Girardeau
Jefferson City

Lee's Summit
Springfield
St. Joseph
St. Louis

Mississippi
Jackson
Tupelo

Montana
Billings
Helena

North Carolina
Asheville
Charlotte
Gastonia
Greensboro
Greenville
Raleigh (2)
Salisbury
Wilmington

North Dakota
Bismark
Fargo

Nebraska
Columbus
Lincoln
Omaha

New Hampshire
Portsmouth

New Jersey
Deptford
East Brunswick
Fair Lawn
Toms River
Hamilton
Union (2)
Verona

New Mexico
Albuquerque

Nevada
Las Vegas (2)
Reno

New York
Albany
Amherst
Brooklyn Heights (2)
East Syracuse
Garden City
Ithaca
Melville (2)
Manhasset
Midtown (3)
New York City
Penn Plaza (3)
Queens/Rego Park
Rochester
Staten Island
Vestal
Wappingers Falls
Watertown
White Plains

Ohio
Akron
Centerville
Cincinnati (2)
Columbus
Hillard
Lima
Mentor
Niles
Reynoldsburg
Strongsville
Toledo

Oklahoma
Oklahoma City
Tulsa

Oregon
Eugene

Milwaukie
Portland

Pennsylvania
Allentown
Clarks Summit
Erie
Harrisburg
Lancaster
North Wales (2)
Philadelphia
Pittsburgh (2)
York

Rhode Island
Cranston

South Carolina
Charleston
Greenville
Myrtle Beach
Irmo

South Dakota
Sioux Falls

Tennessee
Chattanooga
Clarksville
Franklin
Knoxville
Madison
Memphis (2)

Texas
Abilene
Amarillo
Arlington
Austin
Beaumont
Bedford
Corpus Christi
El Paso
Houston
Kingwood
Lubbock
Mesquite
Midland
New Braunfels
San Antonio
Sugar Land (2)
Tyler
Waco

Utah
Odgen
Orem
Salt Lake City

Virginia
Fairfax (2)
Lynchburg
Mechanicsville
Newport News
Roanoke

Vermont
Williston

Washington
Mountlake Terrace (2)
Puyallup
Spokane

Wisconsin
Fox Point
Madison
New Berlin
Racine

West Virginia
Morgantown
S. Charleston

Wyoming
Casper

Puerto Rico
Hato Rey

Virgin Islands
St. Croix

Bibliography

American College of Sports Medicine: <u>ACSM's Guidelines for Exercise Testing and Prescription</u>, Sixth Edition, Lippincott Williams & Wilkins, 2000

American Heart Association: <u>BLS for Healthcare Providers</u>, American Heart Association, 2001

Anderson D: <u>Mosby's Medical, Nursing, and Allied Health Dictionary</u>, Sixth Edition, Mosby, Inc., 2002

Arnheim D: <u>Essentials of Athletic Training</u>, Third Edition, Mosby-Year Book, Inc., 1995

Bickley L, Szilagyi P: <u>Bates' Guide to Physical Examination and History Taking</u>, Eighth Edition, Lippincott Williams & Wilkins, 2003

Bly L: <u>Motor Skill Acquisition in the First Year</u>, Therapy Skill Builders, 1994

Brannon F, Foley M, Starr J, Saul L: <u>Cardiopulmonary Rehabilitation: Basic Theory and Application</u>, F.A. Davis Company, 1998

Brunnstrom S: <u>Movement Therapy in Hemiplegia</u>, Harper and Row Publishers Inc., 1970

Buchanan L, Nawoczenski D: <u>Spinal Cord Injury: Concepts and Management Approaches</u>, Williams & Wilkins, 1987

Cameron M: <u>Physical Agents in Rehabilitation: From Research to Practice</u>, W.D. Saunders Company, 1998

Campbell S: <u>Decision Making in Pediatric Neurologic Physical Therapy</u>, Churchill Livingstone, 1999

Campbell S: <u>Physical Therapy for Children</u>, Second Edition, W.B. Saunders Company, 2000

Ciccone C: <u>Pharmacology in Rehabilitation</u>, Third Edition, F.A. Davis Company, 2002

Clark C, Bonfiglio M: <u>Orthopaedics: Essentials of Diagnosis and Treatment</u>, Churchill Livingstone, 1994

Currier D: <u>Elements of Research in Physical Therapy</u>, Second Edition, Williams & Wilkins, 1984

Davis C: Patient Practitioner Interaction, Third Edition, Slack Inc., 1998

De Domenico G, Wood E: Beard's Massage, W.B. Saunders Company, 1997

Ellis D, Lamkowitz S, Maisey-Ireland M: Master Student, College Survival Inc., 1986

Frownfelter D, Dean E: Principles and Practice of Cardiopulmonary Physical Therapy, Third Edition, Mosby-Year Book, Inc., 1996

Garrison S: Physical Medicine and Rehabilitation Basics, J.B. Lippincott Company, 1995

Giles S: A Guide to Success: Physical Therapist Assistant's Review for Licensure, Mainely Physical Therapy, 2002

Giles S, Stuart J: Test Master: Physical Therapist Assistant Examination, Mainely Physical Therapy, 2003

Goodman C, Boissonnault W: Pathology: Implications for the Physical Therapist, W.B. Saunders Company, 1998

Goodman C, Snyder T: Differential Diagnosis in Physical Therapy, Third Edition, W.B. Saunders Company, 2000

Goold G: First Aid in the Workplace, Prentice-Hall, 1995

Gross J, Fetto J, Rosen E: Musculoskeletal Examination, Second Edition, Blackwell Science, Inc., 2002

Guide for Conduct of the Physical Therapist Assistant, American Physical Therapy Association, 2001

Guide to Physical Therapist Practice, Second Edition, American Physical Therapy Association, 2001

Haggard A: Handbook of Patient Education, Aspen Publishers, 1989

Hamill J, Knutzen K: Biomechanical Basis of Human Movement, Williams & Wilkins, 1995

Hertling D, Kessler R: Management of Common Musculoskeletal Disorders, Third Edition, Lippincott, 1996

Hickock R: Physical Therapy Administration and Management, Williams & Wilkins, 1982

Hillegass E, Sadowsky H: Cardiopulmonary Physical Therapy, 2nd Edition, WB Saunders, Inc., 2001

Hoppenfeld S: Physical Examination of the Spine and Extremities, Appleton-Century-Crofts, 1976

Irwin S, Tecklin J: Cardiopulmonary Physical Therapy, Third Edition, Mosby-Year Book, Inc., 1995

Kendall F, McCreary E, Provance P: Muscle Testing and Function, Williams & Wilkins, 1993

Kettenbach G: Writing S.O.A.P. Notes, Second Edition, F.A. Davis Company, 1995

Kisner C, Colby L: Therapeutic Exercise Foundations and Techniques, Fourth Edition, F.A. Davis Company, 2002

Levangie P, Norkin C: <u>Joint Structure and Function: A Comprehensive Analysis</u>, Third Edition, F. A. Davis Company, 2001

Long T, Toscano K: <u>Handbook of Pediatric Physical Therapy</u>, Second Edition, Lippincott Williams & Wilkins, 2002

Magee D: <u>Orthopedic Physical Assessment</u>, Fourth Edition, W.B. Saunders Company, 2002

Michlovitz S: <u>Thermal Agents in Rehabilitation</u>, Third Edition, F.A. Davis Company, 1996

Minor M, Minor S: <u>Patient Care Skills</u>, Fourth Edition, Appleton & Lange, 1999

<u>National Physical Therapy Examinations Candidate Handbook</u>, Federation of State Boards of Physical Therapy, 2002

Norkin C, White D: <u>Measurement of Joint Motion: A Guide to Goniometry</u>, Edition Two, F.A. Davis Company, 1995

O'Sullivan S, Schmitz T: <u>Physical Rehabilitation: Assessment and Treatment</u>, Fourth Edition, F.A. Davis Company, 2001

Pauls J, Reed K: <u>Quick Reference to Physical Therapy</u>, Aspen Publishers, 1996

Paz J, Panik M: <u>Acute Care Handbook for Physical Therapists</u>, Butterworth-Heinemann, 1997

Pierson F: <u>Principles and Techniques of Patient Care</u>, Second Edition, W. B. Saunders Company, 1999

Purtilo R, Haddad A: <u>Health Professional and Patient Interaction</u>, Sixth Edition, W. B. Saunders Company, 2002

Ratliffe K: <u>Clinical Pediatric Physical Therapy: A Guide for the Physical Therapy Team</u>, Mosby, 1998

Robinson A, Snyder-Mackler L: <u>Clinical Electrophysiology</u>, Williams & Wilkins, 1995

Rothstein J, Roy S, Wolf S: <u>The Rehabilitation Specialist's Handbook</u>, F.A. Davis Company, 1998

Saunders H, Saunders R: <u>Evaluation, Treatment and Prevention of Musculoskeletal Disorders</u>, Third Edition, Volume One Spine, The Saunders Group, 1993

Scott R: <u>Promoting Legal Awareness in Physical and Occupational Therapy</u>, Mosby, Inc., 1997

Shamus E, Shamus J: <u>Sports Injury: Prevention & Rehabilitation</u>, McGraw-Hill Companies, Inc., 2001

<u>Standards of Ethical Conduct for the Physical Therapist Assistant</u>, American Physical Therapy Association, 2001

<u>Standards of Practice for Physical Therapy</u>, American Physical Therapy Association, 2002

Starkey C, Ryan J: <u>Evaluation of Orthopedic and Athletic Injuries</u>, F.A. Davis Company, 1996

Sullivan P, Markos P: <u>Clinical Procedures in Therapeutic Exercise</u>, Appleton and Lange, 1996

Sultz H: <u>Health Care USA: Understanding Its Organization and Delivery</u>, Second Edition, Aspen Publishers, 1999

Umphred D: <u>Neurological Rehabilitation</u>, Fourth Edition, Mosby, Inc., 2001

Walter J: <u>Physical Therapy Management</u>, Mosby, Inc., 1993

Waxman S, deGroot J: <u>Correlative Neuroanatomy</u>, Appleton & Lange, 1995

| **Examination Preparation**

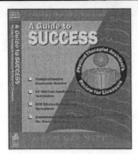 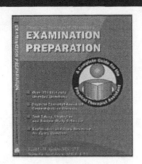 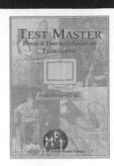